HANDS ON

of related interest

Queer Sex
A Trans and Non-Binary Guide to
Intimacy, Pleasure and Relationships
Juno Roche
ISBN 978 1 78592 406 4
eISBN 978 1 78450 770 1

Written on the Body
Letters from Trans and Non-Binary Survivors
of Sexual Assault and Domestic Violence
Lexie Bean
ISBN 978 1 78592 797 3
eISBN 978 1 78450 803 6

Trans Love
An Anthology of Transgender
and Non-Binary Voices
Freiya Benson
ISBN 978 1 78592 432 3
eISBN 978 1 78450 804 3

HANDS ON

Stories of Sexuality Work, Intimacy and Healing

EDITED BY
REMI NEWMAN

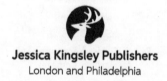

Jessica Kingsley Publishers
London and Philadelphia

First published in Great Britain in 2025 by Jessica Kingsley Publishers
An imprint of John Murray Press

2

Lyrics in chapter 18 are from 'The Lady In Red'
Words and Music by Chris De Burgh Copyright © 2002 BMG Rights Management
(UK) Ltd. All Rights Administered by BMG Rights Management (US) LLC All Rights
Reserved Used by Permission
Reprinted by Permission of Hal Leonard LLC

This book contains mention of abuse, drugs and sex.

A CIP catalogue record for this title is available from the
British Library and the Library of Congress

ISBN 978 1 83997 870 8
eISBN 978 1 83997 871 5

Printed and bound in Great Britain by Clays Ltd

Jessica Kingsley Publishers' policy is to use papers that are natural, renewable
and recyclable products and made from wood grown in sustainable forests.
The logging and manufacturing processes are expected to conform to the
environmental regulations of the country of origin.

Jessica Kingsley Publishers
Carmelite House
50 Victoria Embankment
London EC4Y 0DZ

www.jkp.com

John Murray Press
Part of Hodder & Stoughton Ltd
An Hachette Company

The authorised representative in the EEA is Hachette Ireland,
8 Castlecourt Centre, Dublin 15, D15 XTP3, Ireland (email: info@hbgi.ie)

CONTENTS

INTRODUCTION

Write the story no one knows. This was the advice I gave to two sex workers. I had asked each to write a vignette for a human sexuality university textbook. They were colleagues of mine and I knew they had something powerful to share.

What I received were two poignant stories full of insight and compassion. Daddy Lance, an escort and surrogate partner, shared the story of working with a man who was at the end of his life. He wrote, "I am crying as I write this." At that point I was crying too.

Natasha Strange, a pro-domme, told how although she didn't fit the stereotype of a dominatrix, she was skilled at her job. Her greatest asset, she wrote, was her compassion.

This is a side of sex work we don't often hear about—the immense potential for compassion and healing. I knew there had to be other stories like this. That is how the idea for *Hands On* was born.

As professionals in the field of human sexuality, we can do a lot to help people grow and find a deeper understanding of their sexuality, but there are times when some hands-on attention is needed.

In these stories, you will hear examples of people finding the safety they needed to relax and let themselves feel pleasure and intimate connection, sometimes for the first time. In "Gary: My Military Man," Tracy Lee finally finds the magic words to help her client when she says "Soldier, you are off duty" and he is able to be vulnerable, release some of his own pain and cry in her arms.

Mehdi tells a compelling story in "The Case of Sophia D." of helping a client heal from sexual abuse, reclaim her sexuality and ask for what she wants from a partner.

Don Shewey, author of the book *Daddy Lover God*, shares a powerful experience in "The End of Eugene." He is invited to give a tantric massage to a man with amyotrophic lateral sclerosis (ALS). It turns out he had shared many sessions with this same man 15 years earlier and helped him come to terms with his sexuality.

Many of the stories tell of client relationships that happened over several sessions, taking time to build trust, safety and erotic energy. JoJo Bear's story, "His Scars are My Scars," highlights this beautifully, as he shares the gradual unfolding of a deep connection with a client who struggled with body image due to burn scars.

And there is complexity in the giving. e.b. cotenord's stories of her work as an escort showcase this as she talks of emotional exhaustion and depletion of empathy reserves. Giving everything, even just for an hour or two, is not without consequence. She speaks of digging deep to find that part of a person that makes them worthy of love.

A different sort of complexity is illustrated beautifully in "Sex Worker, Heal Thyself," by A.M. Ament. They seamlessly weave stories of being a sex worker with the experience of receiving the services of a sex worker and the intricacies of this relationship, in their own healing journey.

There is one story that doesn't exactly fit the "hands on" theme: "Bush for Sale," by BD White. It does not include any direct touch between client and worker, but there is a connection that is made—an offering—that brings some needed comfort.

Hands On highlights stories of a myriad of sex workers, including escorts, surrogate partners, pro-dommes and sexological bodyworkers. You will hear in these stories how touch ranges from affectionate to loving to hot and erotic, and everywhere in between.

These stories show, through personal narrative, that all forms of sex(uality) work have the potential to provide powerful healing and create a site of compassion and knowing the body. Whether the goal of the work is to titillate and excite, to give sexual pleasure and release, to help someone learn sexual skills and experience intimacy, or to help someone feel good in their body and embrace their sexuality, sex workers play critical roles in the field of human sexual development.

As contributors to this anthology, our hope is that this work is seen as not only valid, but respected and honored.

Many people find it hard to believe that anyone would choose to do sex work. They imagine it is only done for survival reasons or people are forced into it. Yes, there are people who do sex work because they feel they have no other option and some are forced into it, but we must be careful not to conflate all sex workers into these categories.

One of our authors, Emme Witt-Eden, in an email exchange with me, wrote about this, specifically around bondage, discipline, dominance, submission and sadomasochism (BDSM) work. According to Witt-Eden:

> Education is crucial to disentangle consensual sex work from trafficking and coercive labor. Many sex workers operate successful businesses and report higher life satisfaction as a result. By highlighting the agency and empowerment many sex workers feel they have when doing their jobs, we can hopefully reduce societal stigma. Moreover, educating the public about the therapeutic benefits clients receive from sex work, including through pro-BDSM sessions, can help diminish the shame associated with seeking such professional services.
>
> We must decriminalize sex work. When sex work is criminalized, it fosters a hazardous and detrimental environment for both providers and clients. Clients may feel emboldened to threaten providers if their demands aren't met. Moreover, the stigma associated with illegal work can lead clients to disrespect or harm providers. It may seem paradoxical that clients who patronize sex workers would belittle them for their profession, but some clients project their own shame onto the sex worker, often because they feel bad about paying for illegal services. Transactional sexual services, when conducted consensually between adults, hold no inherent moral wrongdoing, especially considering the benefits clients can derive from such sessions.

In communications with me, Fariba Arabghani, another one of our authors in this book, wrote about the history of the connection between sexuality and spirituality and how sex workers were once held in high esteem in many cultures around the world. She connected this history with the struggle today.

Despite the challenges posed by legal and societal stigma, many in the sex work community continue to provide essential support and healing to their clients, embodying the compassionate core that has always been at the heart of this work.

The legacy of sacred sex work informs current advocacy efforts, emphasizing the dignity, rights and safety of sex workers. Across the globe, sex workers and their allies are fighting for decriminalization, legal reforms and societal acceptance, striving to create a world where sex work is acknowledged as a legitimate and valuable form of labor.

Arabghani wanted us to reconsider our contemporary views on sex work, which will challenge us to:

recognize the complex humanity, dignity and potential for healing that lies at its core. By reflecting on the ancient practices of sacred sex work, we can draw inspiration for a more compassionate, understanding approach to sex work today. A future that honors the holistic, healing dimensions of sexuality and recognizes the invaluable contributions of sex workers to our collective well-being and spiritual growth is within our reach. Through education, advocacy and a renewed appreciation for the sacredness of sexuality, we can bridge the gap between the ancient and modern, fostering a world that respects and uplifts the legacy of the divine in sex work.

It is important to acknowledge that many sex workers experience high levels of discrimination and violence. This is especially true for those working on the street. In the United States, it is Black and Brown transgender sex workers who are at highest risk for violence. It is critical that we aid in the decriminalization movement for sex workers' rights and safety. Part of the proceeds from *Hands On* will be donated to organizations that directly support sex workers.

Remi Newman

Editor's note: In each story, names and details have been changed in order to protect the identity of the clients.

CHAPTER 1
HIS SCARS ARE MY SCARS

JoJo Bear

Early on in my career as a novice "sex guide" I was working in a dusty ramshackle of a place in Berkeley near the Ashby Bart Station. The space housed a clunky mix of bodyworkers, sex practitioners, coaches and other misfits doing some really important work. I graduated from a sexological bodywork program about four years before that, which trained me in using one-way touch with clients. I quickly realized that most of the people I worked with as clients did not know how to touch other people. My work had to be two-way touch.

My eager yet wispy commitment to helping others who were stuck erotically became a practice of learning on the job. Although I had learned some methods from teachers in the past, I sensed I couldn't stick to a script. I was eager to discover and develop my style. I saw plenty of men who needed help with erectile difficulties, mostly from watching too much porn, being too cerebral, being sexual with another person, or simply because of age.

It was the same thing over and over again and I tried my best to get these dudes into their bodies using everything from discovering their erotic core theme, introducing them to the wheel of consent, breathwork, and even dancing around naked.

I tried it all: wrestling, role-play, domination, erotic hypnosis...but something shifted when I met Sid (not his real name).

Sid's first email was brief and simple.

He wrote: *I have body issues, can you help me?*

I replied that of course I could.

That is what I was waiting for, someone I could help with something so close to my heart—my struggles with my skin.

I didn't hear back from Sid for three months, then he called me on the phone for a consultation. He told me that he had not had sex or even touched another person due to his body issues.

I asked all the professional questions regarding his body, but he was pretty mum.

He said, "I had an injury a decade ago." That was it. I decided not to press the issue. Meanwhile, my insecure practitioner mind was spinning. Did I not do the right intake? Was I already handling this badly? However, part of me was trusting him and his process.

He arrived on one of those damp and rainy evenings that happen in the San Francisco Bay Area. The building was quiet and empty of any other people because it was a late weekday evening. It would just be us.

When I entered the waiting room, I was surprised to see a very attractive man in his early fifties. He didn't appear to have any injury, weight issues, an odd walk, a wheelchair or a cane. I immediately wondered if this was the guy I was expecting.

I was stumped, but we both walked into my studio and sat down. Then he told me his story.

About ten years earlier he had been in a house fire. About 80 percent of his body was burned. His face and hands were not harmed. His tone of voice sounded wooden and clinical. I imagined that he had recited this story over and over to nurses, surgeons and physicians.

I noticed my desire to ask him so many questions, but I did not interrupt. I just listened.

I saw how he hid his scars underneath his pants and long-sleeved shirt. And I was keenly aware that I had done the same thing years before.

Shortly thereafter he revealed that he had not been touched by anyone in ten years. He told me that only surgeons or medical doctors had touched his skin. He had not had any intimate contact with anyone in ten years.

His voice and his body went from wooden to animated when he said the words *ten years*.

Again, he asked if I could help. With some heaviness in my throat, I said yes.

After all, hadn't I felt the same fears? Hadn't I avoided any intimate contact from others, just as Sid had done?

I have psoriasis, an immune system disease that creates inflammation inside the body and on the skin. Its causes are unclear, but it appeared when I was a kid, at first as just visible patches on my skin that came and went. When I reached adulthood, it spread all over my body. TV commercials talk about the heartbreak of psoriasis, and I know exactly what they mean.

I spent days, sometimes weeks, alone without being touched.

I was living and working in Los Angeles where the sidewalks were filled with scantily clad folks, but I clothed myself from head to toe. In isolation, hiding and grieving. I walked the same streets contemplating suicide.

Fortunately, I was prescribed medication that helped manage my symptoms. But some emotional scars never left me.

And here was Sid, right in front of me.

During our initial sessions, we did trust-building practices, using touch while fully clothed, establishing agreements and fostering rapport with each other. I noticed the different hats I wore: friend, brother, lover, gay mother, father. I saw Sid be silly, playful, funny. This was evidence of a growing trust; it made my heart flutter.

That's when I introduced and explained a "witnessing" practice. In this ritual, Sid could reveal and talk about his body. He could take off as little or as much clothing as he chose, while describing his relationship to his body. We agreed to use the language of consent and the freedom to change your mind at any time. I explained that, during the practice, I would look only at his eyes until he asked me to look elsewhere. Sid had full agency in the process. This would give him the experience of being seen.

He declined the witnessing ritual instantly, but during our next session, Sid quietly sat in deep thought.

I mirrored him.

Then he leaned forward and looked directly into my eyes: "I want to show you my body, I really do, but I am terrified!"

We sat in silence for a bit.

I took a deep breath, mirroring his body language by leaning forward and saying, "I'll go first!" That meant Sid would be the witness and stay clothed while I undressed.

I stood up and said, "Sid, would *you* mind holding space for me while I talk to you about my body?"

He nodded.

"Would you be willing to sit over there?" I pointed to a chair that was about a foot away from the one he was in.

"Yes!" he said, and he moved to that chair.

I still smile when recalling his boyish excitement as he switched seats.

I looked at him and said, "You can ask me any question. Seriously, anything you want to know about my body, feel free to ask."

I undressed completely.

I'd done this ritual before but the energy had never felt this heightened. I felt an intense desire to protect him. I wanted to be cautious and honor the safe container we had created. I reminded myself that I was doing this for him. I was mindful to not complain about my body in front of Sid. I felt so protective of him and I trusted whatever was happening at this moment.

His eyes darted all over my body. I said things like, "I really love my beard, my teeth are amazing, it's a family thing, I don't really do much with them, but I do brush them!"

"I love that I am hairy. When I get out of a pool I like to dance around and shake my body like a wet dog. Even my cock and balls flop around."

I looked down at my crotch and joked, "Oh yeah, there they are!" He smiled, and started to giggle.

He asked me safe, generic questions at first. My role was to give short answers and help Sid track his body. I hoped he'd ask about my skin because that's the issue that led him here. At first, he asked "safe" questions such as, "How did you get that scar on your wrist?" My answer was intentionally short. "It is from a fight I had when I was 26." He asked about my weight and I said, "I struggle with it."

I appreciated his interest and enthusiasm. He was buying into the practice.

In a silly voice I said, "This is your session, you know. I want to make sure you can take a turn—if you choose."

He nervously said, "I am ready!"

"Are you sure?" I looked into his eyes.

"Yes!" he nodded.

I started to lean over and pick up my clothing to put it back on, but he asked, "Could you stay undressed?"

I felt warm in my body, excited by seeing him take charge.

I smiled and said, "Sure. Where do you want me to sit?"

"Right where you are standing." He stood up and brought me his chair (even though my chair and clothing were closer to me). As the practitioner, Sid's eagerness and attention demonstrated a major shift in his experience. He was now trusting the practice and was excited about it.

As a human being, I felt a wave of shyness come over me as I experienced his gift of care.

I thanked him, put my clothes on the chair, and sat.

As I watched him stand in front of me in that dark musty room I saw his hands shake slightly, his eyes staring right into mine. I heard his breath. I no longer heard the rain outside the window. I heard only him. I felt as if we were the only two people in the world. Everything went quiet.

Softly, he talked for a while about his face, ears, eyes and hair (he had a nice head of hair).

Some things he repeated. My inner guide wondered if he was stalling so he wouldn't have to disrobe.

I reminded myself to meet him where he was in that moment. None of this was a race. He'd had ten years of not wanting to show anyone his body.

I reminded him that I would only look at his eyes unless he

instructed me otherwise. He replied, "You can look wherever you want." This was significant.

"I think I am ready to unbutton my shirt," he announced. It felt like a warning.

As he shakily removed his top, he exposed his scars from the fire. He clutched his shirt closely, I sensed he was feeling vulnerable. His body language suggested he was cold, although the room was warm. A long stretch of quietness inhabited the room.

I took a deep breath in the silence.

I looked slowly at his chest, torso, belly, forearms and shoulders. I did not stare too long. My job was to witness, not expose, so I kept bringing my eyes back to his eyes.

He softly said, "I miss this hairy chest." His fingers lightly grazed the scars all over his chest. He talked about the difference between his former body and its current state. He referred to the fire as the incident. "Before the incident I loved to hook up with a lot of men. I enjoyed how my body could give others so much pleasure."

He was entering the zone where his history was a vivid beam of light illuminating the room.

He talked about a cruisy beach in Italy, a year before the "incident," where he met local men who did not speak any English. But they did manage to kiss every part of his body. I watched him share this memory of embodied pleasure. And I saw how it was interrupted as he realized where he was now.

He got quiet and small.

I imagined the sadness and anguish he was feeling at that moment.

Time seems to stop when I hold space for another. It's

perplexing but somewhat reassuring when I participate in something sacred. I realize how ostentatious that may sound. Still, I recall a mentor saying that people who do sex work are priestesses and priests who wear fewer costumes.

When Sid went quiet, I asked if he wanted me to ask him questions.

He said yes.

"Does it hurt?" I asked.

"Most of it is numb," he replied. "I don't feel much sensation when I touch my scars."

He then reminded me, "I have only been touched by medical professionals!"

Silence.

"Would you like me to touch you?" I asked.

He looked at me for a long time, still clutching his shirt with one hand.

I started judging myself, thinking *Did I say something wrong?*

Here is what I did say: "You are still in charge. Would you like to do something, like take my hand and place it wherever you want?"

Sid put down his shirt and stepped closer to me.

He grabbed my hand and placed it over his heart. I wanted to cry but I held it in and took a deep breath with him.

"What do you notice?" I asked.

"I feel the warmth of your hand. It feels good!" he whispered.

He then moved my hand to his very scarred belly. I felt its little ridges and roughness. I felt as if my hand was touching a canvas of acrylic painting. I continued looking into his eyes.

He stared down at my hand on his body. He then stared into my eyes. "I like your belly."

He turned away with a nervous smile.

Then he said, "Really?"

"Yes, I am a fan of bellies!" I said. "May I put my belly against yours?"

He nodded and again I saw that boy again who brought me the chair. There was excitement in his face.

I stood up, lifted my hand away from his body and leaned my belly into his. I took a deep breath to help him remember to breathe.

He did.

He closed his eyes, swayed a little so his scarred belly was grazing my hairy belly. He looked into my eyes. "Can I wrap my arms around you?" he said. His voice much deeper now, a sign of a shift occurring in his mind and spirit.

I smiled and said, "Of course!"

He pulled me tightly and our bellies and chests were connected. He enveloped me in his embrace. I felt his body soften, let go and become aroused. His breath was stronger and he had an erection.

We stayed in the embrace while I waited for Sid to make the first move.

Because of his height his cheek rested near my eye. He started to weep.

His hard, guttural cry sounded powerful enough to reach across the bay.

I felt his tears roll down my face, some probably mixed with mine. We stayed that way for a long time. He grabbed his t-shirt to blow his nose. "Whoa," I said. "I have Kleenex for that!"

We lay chest to chest for the rest of the session.

He didn't remove any more clothing as we kept cuddling,

and as the session closed and he gathered himself, I noticed how elastic his body was. His shoulders were relaxed; he was animated and boyish.

I was so proud of him.

I felt love for him at that moment.

I can use my scars to serve other people's scars.

CHAPTER 2

THE COST; STRINGS OF LIES; COLD HEART CASH

e.b. cotenord

THE COST

Scene: A woman walks down a wet sidewalk in the night. Her stilettos pierce the puddles like Olympic divers, barely a splash. A wig brushes the rims of her large black sunglasses, and her red lips are the only distinguishable facial feature as she passes in front of a red neon sign and into the glow of a luxury hotel. Her trench hits mid-calf, collar turned up. As she enters the elevator, she adjusts the lace that's strapping stockings to her thighs underneath.

She exits the elevator. The shot, the movement, the layout of the scene perfectly mirror the scene of a prisoner being escorted to his cell in another story. Different wardrobe. Different lighting. Different finishes on the walls and floors and doorways. But the walk, the desolation as she steps toward a destiny of isolation in a small room, are exactly the same. Her handcuffs are metaphorical, the guards leading her down the hall are her bills, and her fear of returning to her previous life is her cell.

She takes a deep breath, exhales and shakes her shoulders and face gently to ensure the remnants of her human persona are entirely brushed off as she folds her manicured acrylic nails into her palm to gently tap the door with her knuckles. The audience hears the doorknob and the creak of the hinge as the door cracks open as far as the chain will allow.

The shot freezes and a voice or a title-card presents itself to the viewer, promising that the rewards for entering the room are great but "at what cost?"

The viewer is intrigued by this dilemma. The question of whether they would risk it all rolls around in their mind.

"Would I?"

"What would it take?"

"Would it be worth it?"

"Could I risk it all?"

And while others are intrigued by the question itself, I'm intrigued by the implication of the premise. I don't deny that the cost of walking into that room is enormous. I know precisely what that cost is. It's not paid as I enter one room or individual rooms, it's a tab that is run up over years of being in the business. It's definitive. It's quantifiable. It's social and political. It's personal. But for the civilians indulging in experimental thought sex trade voyeurism, the cost is an estimation of the net totals of their fantasies and shame.

We cut from the scene and its cliches and tropes and we're left with me, playing a role, in a fantasy that plays out in someone else's reality. The door opens, he smiles. I apologize for being seven minutes late. I'm always seven minutes late. I never take into account valet or the time it takes to call the elevator or the length of the hallways or my inability to accurately read the signs telling me which direction I'm supposed to go to arrive at the correct room number.

I know before I've arrived exactly where the elevators are, how to avoid eye contact with each particular front desk staff. I know if the elevator needs a key. I know the layout of the room and whether they have the *good* robes. I know whether they offer Perrier or San Pellegrino and whether the client will apologize for the hotel only having Perrier when I specifically requested San Pellegrino.

But I don't know how long it's going to take me to get to the room from my car. Except that however long it takes, it will get me there seven minutes late. And so I apologize. The clock starts when I arrive, not when the booking was supposed to begin, and I'm certain he'll forget about those seven minutes in the next 45 seconds or so.

I'm not wearing a wig. Or sunglasses. Or a trench coat. Or anything that screams, "I AM A SPY STEALTHILY SNEAKING INTO YOUR HOTEL AT NIGHT TO COMMIT ILLEGAL ILLICIT ACTS OF DEBAUCHERY!"

My nails are natural and short. I know plenty of my colleagues prefer long nails, and their clients are fans of the look. But I tend to specialize in acts where fingernails are contraindicated. I keep them painted so they look clean. I keep them short to keep marks off flesh, inside and out. I'm in a white dress. Stilettos. Red lipstick. Dressed to make him forget about the seven minutes. To sear the image of my presence into his memory so he spends the next several months imagining the moment he opened the door, to see me standing there ready to risk it all with him.

He is in khakis. He is always in khakis. They are always in

khakis. And an impossible puzzle of a belt. He's also hoping to impress. But I'm more impressed by the extra paper in the envelope. We don't discuss that. I slide it into my purse. He has forgotten about the seven minutes and is now apologizing for the dearth of Pellegrino. And according to the narrator, *this* is the point of no return. The part of the story where we have to weigh the cost of whether what is going to happen next is worth it.

In the scene, she's dressed for the occasion. She arrived. She knocked. She entered the room. She took the cash. Does she go through with it?

The actress playing the part of me would now be directed to act as if she is not intimidated by his confidence and wealth, but she's terrified and uncertain. The gentleman is ready to prey, and she must present as if he is not and as if she is ready and eager to impress, thinly veiling the fact that she is afraid she will not. The lights are dim. She is wide-eyed. She has so much to lose tonight.

I put my bag down on the nightstand, next to the lamp and the phone, open the Perrier and take a sip, marking the green bottle with my red lipstick. I begin the small talk. He's nervous. I am not. I calm him, and yes, I go through with it. The cost, at the moment, is mostly his, a small collection of $100 bills.

The cost of each interaction for me is minimal. The cost is not my dignity, my worth, my sense of self seeping out of my loins as the mounds of my inner thighs fail to hold it all in when I move them apart. I am not selling pieces of myself to men until there is nothing left of me worthy of a sticker, as if one day, my inventory will dwindle down to an earlobe or a wonky toe and then I will no longer have anything to offer.

But I am a surrogate. A woman, but a woman who is here to fulfill the duties of an ideal woman. To complete the tasks that he thinks other women are failing to do for him. And to do it as a complete package, fulfilling the duties other women do as well because it is expected of us. To show up and be a perfect woman. A dream girl—in a way that doesn't feel contrived. It must be authentic. It must connect with him and it must connect with his needs and ideals and fantasies.

I build the heat between our palms as I bring them close together. I read his desires like braille on his skin with my fingers. And the pressure of his lips confesses his needs to me. I watch his face; I navigate and translate each whimper and wince. Is it pain? Is it excitement? Is it shame? Is it fear of the unknown? Fear of getting caught? And are those fears exactly what is bringing him closer to heights that will make him forget them altogether?

Is his wife a disapproving ghost in his head and does he want that ghost to watch in disgust? Is she blissfully unaware and would he be ashamed if such a reputable woman knew about his depravity? He needs to know he's not depraved. That he's decent and acceptable. But he needs to feel that it's in him to be depraved.

He's terrified and I am here to guide him into it, through it and away from it. Or maybe he's not, and I'm supposed to give him a reason to feel guilty and shameful enough to feel pleasure. But I refuse to indulge the fantasy of our time together being shameful, and leave him alone to answer to the glares from his phantom wife silently mouthing her vows in the corner of his mind.

I press my body against his to bring him back to me. I

expand my ribs wide against his torso and exhale. Each breath slow, deliberate, calm. My heart rate is slower than his. I want him to feel the steady rhythms of my body and match them. The thumps of my heart echoed in a call and answer with his. His breath moving deep in unison with mine. To feel his body relaxing while it simultaneously builds excitement. The pressure is disorienting. It's dizzying.

He feels high, he feels heaven, but he looks below us to see a god who would judge us if he could look up and if he weren't too busy consoling a desolate wife. He looks down to realize that down and up and above and below are mechanisms of gravity and the only gravity that still exists in the room is the one pulling our bodies together. Electricity conducted in the sweat and salt of our skin, a buzz and a shock and an energy that cause him to lose the signal to my pulse, the pulse that was dictating his and the flow of blood through his body. His limbs are satellites orbiting my body and crashing.

My attention takes a break while I go on physical autopilot. I'm thinking about this metaphor and comparing blackholes to pink holes and closing my eyes to withhold giggles at the idea of "spaghettification" on being sucked into the hole. One of the expectations of me is to be amusing, but not so amusing I come across as anything more than disarming. I shouldn't be adding much to conversations because I shouldn't be showing up the man. I shouldn't be too comfortable. Too smart. Too dumb. Too awkward. Too confident. Too insecure. I must keep his masculinity in balance with my femininity in ways that he expects and exactly how he expects.

I need to allow him to lead the conversations, and I follow along. I need to allow him to finish my jokes. I will be interesting and intelligent if I keep my mouth shut, but only in the right amount. Only in exactly the right proportions. Too quiet and I'm a bimbo. Too talkative and I'm a bimbo. Too thoughtful and I'm a bitch. Too many jokes and I'm a bitch. If I am impressed by him and interested in him, then I will be impressive and interesting in turn. And I can't make astrophysics jokes while he's attempting to make these 187 seconds of disappointing missionary into the quantum psychosexual manifestation of a supernova.

I allow him to believe it is. I encourage him to believe it. I actively engage in the fantasy that he is an experience that is indescribable given the limitations of language and modern science. I wish I could talk to his disapproving ghost wife and ask her why she would be upset that I took this chore off her list for her. At the end of our time, there is awkward small talk, and me not-too-explicitly-disagreeing with his often misguided musings about the world and human beings.

But what is the cost? What is the sacrifice? Have I risked it all to have this exchange? The cost isn't that I left my goodness and legacy on the mattress at a three-and-a-half-star hotel. It's not that I felt the sweat of a patent attorney from New Jersey.

The narrator at the door of this room would have you believe that was it. I walked out and I left it all, my soul and my dignity, captured in the lipstick stains on the linens and forever trapped in the walls of that room. And the room itself a ghost in my mind, haunting my dreams indefinitely, and destroying potential.

But it's not. I shower and bid adieu to my client's demons when I leave the room. What's left is the weight of womanhood.

When I leave the room, the expectations of me are not less. They are more. If I can give that much to my clients, physically, mentally and emotionally, then the demand is that I give more to my family, my partner, my friends. I can be quieter and make them more interesting. I can let them finish my jokes so they think I am funny enough to be around. I can show up sexually and emotionally.

In return, they will ask less of me than my clients. They won't expect me to look nice, because that's not actually attractive. They don't expect me to fake pleasure in bed because they're really interested in my pleasure. I am expected to bring genuine pleasure because that pleases them. They don't expect me to carry on conversations or be interesting or gregarious or likable because that's just a fake version of me.

If I can accept a stranger's lies, it would be hypocrisy not to accept them at home. And if I can read a stranger's soul and if I can be a dream girl for a stranger for one hour, how can I not do that and be that when I come home? But not in the dream girl way that my partner thinks my client wants. The dream girl way that my partner wants. The dream girl that is actually not that great, and knows it.

If I can put up with a stranger's lies for hours for money, I should be willing to offer the same to my partner for love. If I can listen to a stranger's stories and explanations of my own experiences, I understand that my partner can do it so much better. If I can be willing to give the best fake parts of me to strangers, I can give those same parts, genuinely, to the people in my life.

And I can.

One of the things I believe is that every person in the world, no matter how deplorable or unlikable, is worthy of love and has lovable traits about them. When I enter into a room with a client, I dig as hard and deep as I can, sometimes twisting myself, to find that thing. To pull it out of them. To make them feel like that part of them is being revered. To honor the divinity of that part of them that they deserve to have honored. I want them to feel as if they matter. Because mattering is the most important experience a human being can have. People will choose to die in an effort to matter. To be martyrs. To stand for a cause. To leave a legacy. Or simply to have meant something important to another person. While each of us has our own ideas about what mattering looks like, we are all driven to matter. We fear never mattering more than we fear death.

I can do that. But the cost of that is emotional exhaustion. The cost of that is at the expense of my empathy reserves. The cost is my social endurance.

The cost of being a whore isn't that I lost a sacred physical connection with others.

The cost of that is that I am angry. I want to matter too. I want the people who see me to see how I matter. I want them to see how I matter in ways that are true and aren't filtered through their own fantasies and expectations that they should get from me what others get. To give others what they get from me, in full, requires that a part of me absolutely resents and hates them for how they treat other people and how much they expect from others.

The cost isn't scarlet monograms and besmirched reputations.

The cost is that my voice and my humanity are disappearing

into lipstick smudges on pillowcases. That the splash-less steps through puddles will leave behind no footprints. That my fingernails won't leave a mark. That no part of me ever will.

STRINGS OF LIES

"You've given me something special. A reason to live."

His eyes, glassy and bloodshot from being day drunk, fill with water as we stand in his condo's parking garage.

I say nothing and brush his lashes with my thumb. Then I run the backs of my fingers down his face, pausing over cheekbones that are too high and too wide for a man so frail. He smiles, and cries.

The valet arrives with my car. The man kisses my hand and places a $200 tip into it. I kiss him goodbye. It's hard to forget being someone's reason to live. He forgot. Or maybe he needed a better reason. Or maybe I just wasn't reason enough. Or maybe he lied.

Lying comes easy to men like him.

After his first bottle of morning wine, he always confessed to me that he was once a lawyer. He would tell me he hated it, how he found the profession unsavory and cruel and hated the person he had to be when he practiced law.

He didn't hate it enough to stop it from making him a millionaire in his forties. And he didn't hate it enough to not still practice law as a hobby in his seventies.

He sips his way through another half bottle while we sit at his table overlooking the harbor 30 floors beneath us. A decorative red envelope with my two-hour fee still sits on the placemat next to my elbow.

"I play the harp," he says. "I love it. I play several hours a day." He tells me he finished his private lesson shortly before I arrived. It might be unfair of me to assume that this is a lie, but I do anyway. He drinks too much to be telling the truth. He couldn't play the harp while shaking in the morning. The amount he would need to drink in order to stop his hands shaking would certainly affect his playing.

"You should play for me some time," I say with a smile. I don't want him to know that I know he never will. I just want to indulge his fantasy. If I can't pretend to find him fascinating, I have no business being here. I am here to make him feel loved and wanted. "I want to hear you play."

I actually did want to hear him play. He was a man who strove for excellence in every area of his life. If he were able to play, he would be extraordinary. I wanted to hear that version of him play the harp, the version of him he thought he was when he'd open his third bottle of wine at 2pm.

At 2pm, I was his reason to live.

It was the one time I believed him. It was the moment I felt an authentic love for him. I held it sacred that I was his reason to live.

But, like the harp, I was nothing more than a fantasy to him. Something he drank too much of to be able to hold on to.

COLD HEART CASH

"You're only in this for the money."

The accusation is lobbed at me by an alcoholic client on the third date, some time after 2am. Sober clients know how to accuse me more diplomatically and with decorum and feigned respect—usually with a comment about how I have a lot of clients and that I probably don't remember them.

"I'm sorry, what was that?" I ask Josh.

I still believe that if I make them repeat what they've just said, the utter stupidity of the statement will sink in. I understand that believing this will ever happen is utterly stupid in and of itself. Of course, I'm in it for the money. It's my fucking job. Why else do people go to work? Sometimes I imagine Josh, and men like him, getting equally as indignant with the pizza delivery driver as they do with me.

"You've been bringing me pizza for two months now. You still want me to pay you? Do you even care about my hunger or are you just in it for the money?"

But even more absurd is that I know this guy just spent half his day on a conference call with Craig from the Cleveland office discussing the granular metrics of the "paradigm shift" and how this affects investors' reactions. I doubt he does this for personal enrichment or because he cherishes his intimate bond with Craig. But now is not the time for indignance or defiance or setting Josh straight. Condescendingly explaining to my client how jobs work is definitely a poor customer service strategy. And there's the practical matter of being alone in a room with a man with substance abuse, impulse control and entitlement issues who is angry with me for coming into his home and tricking him into believing I am a human being. Moments like these are where I earn my money.

I could pretend that I charge so much because I'm exceptionally talented in bed. But I'm not. My clients don't know that. They think I am. But the truth is that they think I'm talented because I charge so much, not the other way around.

That's just marketing and psychology. I'm expensive, and glancing at my price tag, they decide I'm a goddamn angel on earth before I walk in the door. But, let's be honest, it's just a vagina. And my vagina is great and all, but vaginas don't do much on their own and there's only so many things you can do with one. Everything else is just packaging. And my package includes my exquisite emotional diplomacy skills. What I mean is that I'm fairly well-read on child psychology and dog training and that knowledge is comprehensively relevant to managing the tempers and insecurities of drunk naked men.

I don't mean to sound cynical. I'm not dismissive of these men, men like Josh. But I'm not naive. I have to assess and maintain control of every situation. I have to figure out what it is about me wanting money that upsets men like Josh in moments like the one Josh is having right now. Sensing impending danger and responding appropriately is how I've kept my children alive and kept my dogs from eating me. I understand on a fundamental level that we live under heteropatriarchal capitalism and that women's; emotional, sexual and domestic labor is undervalued and exploited. And challenging the status quo by capitalizing on that labor at the expense of socially and economically privileged white men disrupts the hegemony, and that threatens a man's sense of security and challenges the standards of masculinity.

But that's probably not what's upsetting Josh right now while he snorts another line of coke off an issue of *Men's Health* magazine in his River North loft. I mean, it is on a fundamental level, but he thinks it's something else. And I'm going to address that. We can address Josh's masculine existential angst in our next session. Josh doesn't want to hear my theories on how he's been socialized to accept that women should not benefit from sex in a way that leads them towards independence rather than subordination and dependence. And I want Josh to pay me so I can get the fuck out of his apartment in the next eight minutes. So instead of giving him a primer in social radicalization, I look into his glassy twitchy eyes, mentally scanning the muscles of my face to make sure they're relaxed and my "empathetic and caring girlfriend experience" gaze is fully engaged.

"Of course I'm not in it just for the money. Look at us. Look at me. Look at everything we've done and experienced together. Our chemistry. Our bond. Do you think you can buy that?" Yes. Yes, you can. And the craftsmanship and artistry of what he's buying are exceptional. "No one can fake this. I care about you. We're two people here, right now, together. And that's real. The way you make me laugh. The way I make you feel. You know when that's fake. You can't really believe that's not authentic."

That's not entirely untrue. Some clients are easy to like and to enjoy. But I won't allow myself to dislike any of them. My obligation to them is to like them. I'm not looking for a best friend. I'm not looking for a soulmate. I'm here to make this person feel good about himself. So I find the good. I find a way to like them. And when I'm on my game, I figure out what it is they want me to like about them even if that part of them isn't really there. If he wants me to love how creative he is, how funny he is, how powerful he is, I will love that about him. He doesn't have to be those things. He just has to want to be those things. I want him to be those things when he's with me.

"Just because this is my job doesn't mean I don't care about you. It's more than just a job. I love what I do." Actually, I can be pretty indifferent about what I do. I'm really good at it, which

I'm grateful for. I'm not really interested in doing something else for a living, but even if I were, none of the other $500 an hour part-time jobs are ever hiring.

Usually, this conversation never gets repeated. And it satisfies Josh and all the other Joshes enough that they let down their guard and remember that they trust me and that I take excellent care of them physically and emotionally.

The other question I get asked around the third date, regardless of their state of inebriation, is, "Am I weird? Is this weird? Do you think it's weird that I like this?"

This one I can answer honestly, sincerely, empathetically and compassionately. It's maybe the other reason I do this work, or at least find some kind of sense of purpose in it, and the answer is, "No, it is absolutely not weird, and I am so sorry anyone has ever made you feel like it is."

I've learned compartmentalization at a super-human level. How I feel about my clients when I'm at work and how I feel about them at home are separate and they never cross paths. Those feelings do not need to be resolved. That was so hard to come to terms with, but it's an essential survival skill in my profession. I feel for them so deeply in these moments, which makes me loathe them a lot when I get home, but that's another story about another room that I'm not in right now. Right now, I need to ease the conscience of a man turning to me for reassurance that he's not some kind of sexual freakshow.

"Is this weird?" is the moment that I truly feel for my guys.

I know the pain in that question. And I know there is shame in their feelings about being into something vaguely kinky. During the 2016 election, when leaked reports said that Donald Trump hired sex workers to pee on a bed that Obama slept in, the internet couldn't help themselves. Hookers and golden showers are pretty salacious and the world salivated indeed.

My mind—while angry at how my job, which I do with an immense amount of pride and dignity, is scorned and de-humanized—went to thoughts of my clients. The ones who really believe there is something wrong with them for being into golden showers. The truth is, golden showers are vanilla as fuck, and pee is so much less disgusting than pretty much any other bodily fluid encountered during sex. If you let someone put their mouth on your body, anywhere on your body, with all the germs and decaying food from days earlier trapped inside its crevices that only get removed by a doctor once a year and only with special tools, pee should not be where you scoff.

But the world hates "the weird stuff" and these guys have these fantasies and needs. Their fetishes are a part of their sexuality and their sexuality is part of their identity, and the reality is that while they love their wives and their lives with their wives, they fear losing them over wanting and needing to explore their sexuality. It breaks my heart to watch them wrestle with this. And I offer them the space and the boundaries to have that need met. I'll do the weird stuff to them and with them, and when we're done, I'm not interested in interfering with their lives.

When I walk out of that room, the door closes behind me and I disappear from their lives completely until they have me show up again. I keep their secrets with me. They don't have to fear anyone finding out about that-thing-they-like. They can return home, not having to resent their wives for not providing that outlet. I'm not claiming I'm a marriage-saving philanthropist by any means, but I do believe that a person's sexuality and their ability to live that and express that is an important part of their humanity and their happiness.

I'm glad I'm able to do this for my clients. I think it's important that they have someone in their lives who can offer them that. And I'm good at that. I am proud of being able to be good at my job. I'm proud of my ability to command respect while working in a profession that isn't respected by anyone. I'm proud of the fact that I am able to do what I do without internalizing the shame that the world wants me to feel. And that, in turn, my clients don't feel shame for being with me.

But that's a very romanticized explanation of what I do. It's a grind. I go see clients. Admittedly, I try to keep my workload to under five billable hours a week because I'm over 40 years old, and I need a lot of naps to keep up, and I make a pretty good living working five hours a week. But I go in, I do what they need. I become what they need. And then I go home. And I take off my fuck-toy persona and hang it on a hook behind my door and I wash my body of cologne and sweat, and sometimes pee, and whatever else might be on me. And I order Grub Hub and watch Netflix and I count my money. Because that's why I do what I do. It's my job.

SEX WORKER, HEAL THYSELF

A.M. Ament

"Whores are Healers." I read this proclamation scanned across multiple bodies wearing this statement on t-shirts at a sex educator's conference. While joyous for this narrative to be seen, I also knew this was not how all sex workers felt. As a psychotherapist with a sex work history, I saw myself in an intersection that felt congested and difficult to navigate. I approach the word "healer" with caution. Personally and professionally, I feel that "healer" is a verb, an act of love that exists outside your ego and desire for praise. In this theory, you are a healer because someone has experienced you as such. Others' attachment to the experience is outside your control.

My experiences with people who stated close proximity to healing have not always gone well. Massage therapists who dismissed my need for light pressure left bruises across my body. Being diagnosed with multiple psychiatric disorders and undergoing unwanted "treatments" in the service of healing and curing my intersex body, I grew up skeptical of "healers." In my practices, I desire agency with my clients to decide if our work is healing. I was aware that sex work could be healing for some, but historically I struggled with the concept.

When I became a first-time sex buyer in the summer of

2022, I felt isolated, weak and unlovable. I experienced severe reproductive dysphoria on the news surrounding Roe v. Wade. Not having a body that allows for gestation, I experienced flashbacks to medical trauma. Physicians who worried about the structural integrity between my legs. Fear of how my body worked and how it could provide pleasure for a future spouse was discussed when I was around eight years old.

In 2021, I moved from Seattle to New York City where I attempted to study neuroscience to further my research in queer and trans neuronal relationships. In my program, I experienced transphobia, harassment and assault. My work was rejected from any lab research. The shame forced me out of my program and led to active depression. I felt unwanted and a familiar sense of not belonging. My hair fell out and I stopped eating. I found myself "ugly" through the myopia of gender dysphoria and traumas. I did not know how to communicate my experiences to anyone. I had already left a sexually abusive relationship in March 2021 and felt the cumulative disabling impacts being reactivated by complex post-traumatic stress disorder (PTSD). I felt isolated and scared of humans, knowing the pain of interacting with those who harm and being judged by those who saw my experiences as failure. My only links to other people socially were through apps.

I read a post about hiring sex workers to practice intimacy skills and offer support for queer and trans sex workers. This post challenged my relationship to sex work. To me, it was a survival tool, not a therapeutic intervention. When FOSTA/SESTA happened, I wanted to retire as a sex worker. FOSTA/SESTA was the bill, now law, that was allegedly meant to reduce sex trafficking. What it mostly did was impact the ability of sex workers to find work safely. My last clients were a way of saying goodbye to the Craigslist era of fast money through sex work. Yet here I was in New York City, two years after Covid stole intimacy, and I became curious about getting care from a sex worker provider. I knew how to find Johns/clients throughout the years, but I was out of my element in experiencing sex work where I was not the worker. With the disassemblement of swops, Craigslist and Backpage, I did not know where to turn. I relied on the internet to find a worker by googling "How to hire a sex worker."

I found Kai Cheng Thom's amazing article "How do I hire a sex worker?" After browsing independent sex worker websites, I reached out to a non-binary femme who seemed sweet, nerdy and was someone who might give me space to move slowly. Over email I told her I was scared, lonely and wanting to be held. *I can't believe I used to be a hooker*, I thought, as I looked at myself in the mirror. My perceived weakness and ugliness were staring at me, escorting my anxiety back to its monstrosity-like baseline. I was used to the demands of clients, treating me like a fast-food order. I was worried my vulnerability would be seen as not being real, or my demisexuality seen as strange. I did not want to have to explain myself to my worker. I worried about her feelings of safety meeting me, just I had felt in her situations.

I asked her about her boundaries. She told me her limitations with what she could and could not offer. It was good to hear that she knew what her needs were, as I never considered my boundaries much as a worker. Witnessing another worker saying this is what I can and cannot give to you was the first act of healing I felt with her. Healing can look like someone showing you boundaries. Healing can happen as it happens.

After reaching out, I thought about my sex work history. At age 15, it was for places to stay when I was afraid of my violent family. My mantra when Johns got rough with me was "at least it's not being thrown down stairs" or "they are not calling me worthless." Both fractured my body and spirit. Through street community, I learned that I could ask for money for my time and services. Sex work became better as I developed new skills and friends around the Belmont/Clark area of Chicago in the mid 1990s. I learned who the buyers were around the neighborhood, who was safer and who never to go home with. I was able to interpret how men looked at me when walking down the street. Eye contact, which I didn't normally enjoy casually, became a work/survival skill.

Other skills I learned were to have a street name, never carry an ID, but always carry mace and keep a box cutter on you. The list of advice was endless for a young worker, but it kept me safe. I felt as if I had people who cared for me—family—for the first time in my life.

One piece of advice I did not take was "Never let your guard down by doing drugs with the Johns." One John I actually liked as a person offered me Valium. I liked him because he was kind, not demanding. He was the first client I saw for a second time. Younger than other Johns, around mid-twenties, he smelled better than most men and talked to me like a person, holding curiosity and giving me needed emotional attention. When the Valium kicked in during our second session, he was playing an album that was as intoxicating as the pills. "*Souvlaki*," he said when he saw that I was paying close attention to the music. The CD played twice and the Slowdive song I connected with the most was "Alison."

With your talking and your pills/your messed up life still thrills me/Alison I'm lost.

This is who I am, I thought, as my medicated body allowed him inside me without the pain or pressure I associated with penetration. I was enjoying my sexual experience with him, something that I had not felt before in any other sexual experiences. I let him—no, wanted him to—kiss me on the lips, another sex work "no no." I learned from more experienced workers. (It's too intimate, they will think they own you, neck, tits, let them go down on you, but never on the lips, I was told.) Afterwards, he held me and I wanted his closeness. He asked me what my name was. I always used the name "AJ" as it was gender ambiguous and anonymous. "Alison," I said shyly, not sure if he would believe me. "Oh, like the song," he said with a deep pause. "That's your song, Alison." He kissed me deeply. I knew this was not love, or even lust. This was two hurting people holding moments for each other to make the pain less severe, if only for a little bit.

He was lonely; he had lost his girlfriend to "the streets." He told me he couldn't stop using and was afraid of dying. "Not waking up or getting AIDS," he said. "I'd rather just not wake up." He asked me if I was kicked out like the rest of the queer street kids. I was, I left my family because I could not access love from them. Being on the street felt safer than being at "home." He listened and gave me a wonderful experience based on connection and support for both of our pain. I felt that we were good for each other within the parameters of our arrangements. He took out three $20 bills from his wallet as I was getting ready to go. "Take good care, Alison." I never saw him again and neither did any of the other workers around Belmont/ Clark. Like a good shoegaze song, he lived in my experience and slowly faded away, giving me memories of understanding what the components of love were, what love could look like for me in the future.

When I became a sex work client, the pills that Alison adored in the 1990s became a staple of my life. Punk rock years molded my brain to appreciate GABA receptor agonist substances. This class of medications became my saviors when I needed to work and didn't want to. They coddled me through "bad dates" and other assaults. Pills helped me perform and forget in the moment—men who drooled over me, stealthed me and threw me out after they came inside me. A pejorative description of myself at this time may have been "a pill head whore." However, these substances reduced my shame at screaming when I felt unsafe or at fighting for stolen money. These pills made Alison, who gave more of a fight for her life and survival than I could have at that time.

Having been a sex worker over three decades, I knew the culture of the times, the screening questions, what shoes to *not* wear in certain neighborhoods if you didn't want to be picked up for solicitation. I did *not* know how to meet my needs as *a client* of a sex work practitioner. I did not know what to expect.

When I met my worker, I nervously introduced myself. "Hi," I softly muttered, "I'm AJ." She smiled at me with joy in her face. I was not sure what to do next. In all my years as a sex worker, after I learned what to do, I called the shots. Checking to see if someone was a cop, asking for ID, knowing the laws and who the good lawyers were. "So do you want to go for a walk first?" she asked in a relaxed voice and body. She was wearing all black—t-shirt, shorts and high-top chucks, the NYC uniform. She seemed to just be *comfortable*, that vibe seeming mysterious in my experience of being a human.

I recalled my 2000s era of sex work and being on a "girly website." My manager who ran the website had strict guidelines for our appearances. The "little black dress" and heels, and I had to learn to straighten my hair and wear makeup in a structured way. "I want you looking like high-class women, not prostitutes," she told me. I had work guidelines on what topics I was allowed to talk about. When I was at work, I didn't love Cannondale bikes, live music, basset hound puppies or graphic novels. I liked the Sunday *New York Times* crosswords, world politics, took my coffee black and had travel stories I had to recite to my clients. I was performing within a persona and I had to know my lines of this couth version of "Alison."

"So, I'm a former sex worker," I told my worker. I blushed, embarrassed that someone might have heard me on the street. I tried to remember my decision as to why I might have chosen her to practice my intimacy skills. I took a peek at her profile again and the memory came back. Long dark hair, a shy coy smile, a low key "this is who I am" aesthetic, and deep, soft, kind eyes. I chose her the same way I found my first long-term therapist—intuition. I was looking for kindness and to be heard.

I was never sure why people picked me on the street, on the website, or later via Craigslist. I assumed it was for my body. My lush ass, big naturals, and slight hint of ethnic ambiguity. Later on, as I gathered more tattoos, my look gained compliments of "freaky" and assumptions that I "flagged orange," as in "up for anything." You would be surprised how one performs when housing and survival are on the line. One John I worked with during my Craigslist days was enamored with my body, mesmerized by each curve, taking his time touching me with the most loving intentions. I felt myself wet from the attention, affection and appreciation. As a large bodied person, the message I have received most of my life is to make my body and personality smaller for the world to accept me. Johns became known as clients as the world of sex work evolved. For me, my body was slowly becoming a place beloved by many people, including myself. I was evolving too.

When my worker and I made it back to my apartment, we talked while we sat on my couch. It felt similar to an intake appointment as a therapist. My worker could tell I was in no place to make any "first moves" towards any type of intimacy. Normally hyperverbal, I struggled to speak as my anxiety grasped me. My time in New York, Seattle, Chicago, and how fucking sad I was, consumed me.

I felt that someone was paying attention to me, my apartment adornments, my anti-Zionist and pro trans stickers. Somewhere in our preliminary conversation she asked me if I had been bar-mitzvahed. "No," I said casually. "My family said I wasn't worth spending the money on." She looked horrified and within the same moment as hearing her say "Come here," my head was pressed up against her chest in a hug that allowed me to feel the depth of what I had just told her. Instead of being scared by my trauma, it felt as if she wanted to be there with me. With tears still in my eyes, she looked at me and held out her hand. My brain knew this was an invitation. I hesitated for a moment while she patiently waited for me to be ready for touch. After feeling her hand on mine, fingertips dancing on palms, her grip reassuring my safety, she asked if she could kiss me. "Never let them kiss you on the lips" my mind recalled. I ignored this thought.

The next day and throughout the next few weeks, I felt wanted. I had hookups, dressed to show off my body and was able to think about closeness without flashbacks. My mind felt clearer and my anxiety scaled down to allow me to be myself for the first time in two years. I wanted to give her so much credit for how I was feeling after our session.

I saw my worker one more time as a professional, but it didn't feel right. As a demisexual, I did not want sex from her, but the knowledge that healing intimacy and redeveloping my sexuality could happen for me was impactful. Although I felt gratitude, I wanted to play by clinician rules as I was trained to see this work as a service, not as a way to make friends. Saying goodbye was my instinct as our relationship felt like clinical work. However, through boundaries and discussion, we consensually stayed in touch for about a year.

I realized over the year that we maybe didn't like each other as people. I witnessed our personalities change as we saw each other more as ourselves, her slowly showing up as critical, as I was coming out of my shell around her. I wondered if my healing created resentment—an unexpected power dynamic, where I did not need her anymore as my worker. I said to myself "I healed," removing her from any pedestal. *I should have trusted my gut*, I thought, as she eagerly made suggestions on how I should conduct myself socially and directed me to behave in ways she felt she identified as best for me. She was not happy with how I took up space, eerily re-enacting my dynamics with my parents. I was loud, outgoing and happy to be alive—not the person she first met as her client. I fawned, hearing her experiences of me. I did not want to engage with someone who couldn't appreciate me as changed. My confidence was a sign of me becoming closer to myself. The time I spent with my worker was a catalyst for healing, along with reactivating my passion for decriminalization for sex work and drug use.

We are responsible for our own healing. The New Testament proverb "Physician, heal thyself" can be interpreted as take care of your own shit before trying to help anyone else. Through love for myself, I found healing through sex work in various ways. I experienced comfort in touch and with other workers who showed love through resource sharing and caretaking. But the love I feel for myself, which I cultivated through self-respect, is one of my greatest life accomplishments. Having healed as both client and worker through sex work, I have transformed from an unsure and frightened person to someone with confidence and a self-actualized version of myself and my communities and a strong vision about the future of clinical sex work. Sex worker, heal thyself indeed!

THE END OF EUGENE

Don Shewey

Recently, a colleague in Boston passed along an inquiry from a man named Martin, who was looking for someone to give a tantric massage to his partner who has ALS, the degenerative nerve disorder also known as "Lou Gehrig's disease." At first, I said yes, then I realized he was asking me to do an outcall to his partner's home, which ordinarily I don't do. I prefer to work at my own studio with my massage table and other equipment on hand, rather than improvise in somebody else's space. So I declined and suggested my friend Eric, but Eric didn't feel prepared to undertake this assignment. I went back to Martin and said I would do the session, and what was his partner's name? It was only then that I learned we were talking about someone I had done an intense year-long series of sacred intimate sessions with. I'll call him Eugene.

When I met him, Eugene was 44, a handsome Black man, a high-powered entertainment-business executive, married with two children and going through a contentious divorce from his wife while continuing to share a gigantic Upper East Side townhouse. He let me know in our early sessions that he had always had curiosity about sex with men but had suppressed his desires because of social pressure to conform—get married, raise a family, climb the corporate ladder, socialize with other finance bros (skiing in Aspen, pretending to like football, networking at Knicks games). His ideas about sex were equally conventional, pretty much confined to PIV (penis-in-vagina) intercourse-to-ejaculation. Coming to me for erotic massage gave him the opportunity to inhabit the formerly taboo realm of touching and being touched by another man. I introduced him to slow, sensual touch and Body Electric-style breathwork. And I provided a safe space for him to explore mutual oral and anal pleasure, both of which turned out to be revelatory for him. He told me he was dating another woman (to keep up social appearances) and that their sex life had improved noticeably since he started seeing me. He was more relaxed, he could slow down, and he didn't have to be in charge at all times.

He had quaintly amusing straight-guy language for erotic interactions. He appreciated massage but couldn't wait for it to get "interesting." Anything other than penetration he would term "role-playing." Perhaps inevitably, after several sessions, he wondered if it would be possible to have what he called "real sex." As we gravitated from the massage table to the bed, he let me know that he loved kissing, hugging, touching my butt and getting orally serviced. Still, he wondered, "When are we going to go all the way?" In my guise as a somatic sex educator, I made it my mission to spread the gospel of tantra, expanding his notion of what constitutes "real sex," and I clued him in to the principles of safer sex, which emerged from the gay male community during the AIDS epidemic but for the most part escaped the attention of men on the down-low like Eugene. Although he admitted to being a linear thinker, attached to "completion," he agreed to receiving a classic Taoist erotic massage, which combines intense breathing and genital massage with the intention of raising and circulating erotic energy around the body without the goal of ejaculating. He reported finding the experience less erotic than he imagined it would be, yet highly spiritual. The image came to him of being deep in a green medieval forest. He said, "I think I really needed this, but you figured that out, didn't you?"

I loved that Eugene took our sessions seriously. He listened to what I said and thought about it carefully. He was haunted by my asking if anybody else in his life knew that he was attracted to men. He took that as a challenge, and I guess he felt a little defensive. He said it didn't make sense to go public with that admission unless he were in love. Embracing a gay or bisexual identity would mean losing status with his straight male friends and his conservative Southern family. He came to me for pure fun, to escape the rigors of responsibility. I understood and did not require him to make any public declarations.

Inevitably, we did proceed to exploring intercourse with condoms. "Can I do the ultimate?" as he put it. I turned him on to erotic wrestling and using toys (cock rings, dildos and blindfolds) to enhance sexual pleasure. After one climax, he proclaimed, "This is great! It's better than a heavy spiritual trip." I said, "Who says spirit has to be heavy? Spirit dances, too." He heartily agreed, though he fretted that, after these sessions with me, he wouldn't be able to enjoy conventional sex. I said, "Eugene, you never have to have 'conventional sex' again! Bring all of this to your sex partners!" He said that sessions with me did everything he would want a therapy session to do.

After 21 sessions over the course of a calendar year, Eugene called me and wondered if he could take me to dinner to discuss an article I'd shared with him about the Body Electric School and its tantric approach to sexuality. Ordinarily I maintain strict boundaries and don't socialize with clients, but I decided to make an exception this time. I liked Eugene, and if I could encourage him to cultivate more curiosity and self-awareness about his erotic options, I was game. We had a great friendly conversation over an expensive meal, sharing personal histories. But as the dinner was winding down, I realized that Eugene was angling to shift our relationship from client-and-practitioner to something that looked more like dating. It wasn't so much that he wanted to stop paying for sessions—he had plenty of money—but that he was interested in developing a more mutual, interactive emotional connection.

Sex workers face this dilemma with regular clients all the time. If I were younger and hungrier and more adventurous—in other words, if I were a different person—I might have been intrigued to have an affair with a wealthy closeted bisexual businessman, just to see where it would go. But I wasn't a kid anymore, and I didn't think it would be especially rewarding for me or healthy for him. Since he hadn't told anyone else in his life that he was attracted to men, I would be taking on the burden of maintaining his sexual secret. I wanted more for him. I hoped that he would gain the courage and self-confidence to meet other men as peers to explore mutual attraction. And I couldn't help believing that the friends who loved and cared for him would want him to be happy and support him in not hiding. He understood what I was saying, though he felt sad and disappointed. We parted with an affectionate hug, and then I didn't hear from him again.

But then, 15 years later, I got the message from Martin. I was simultaneously delighted to know that Eugene had acquired a male partner and distressed to learn about his illness. Anybody who knows anything about ALS knows that it's a relentless and fatal disease. I looked it up on Wikipedia, which told me that patients are ranked on a Functional Range Scale from 48 (normal and healthy) to zero (incapacitated) and that they lose one point on the scale every month. Survival at three years is 10 percent, a grim prognosis. I've worked with other clients who had severe physical disabilities. I've seen how touch-deprived they tended to be and how much they appreciated receiving even the slightest physical contact. Sad as I was to learn about Eugene's situation, I was willing to provide some pleasure if I could.

It took a few weeks to come up with a date that worked for everyone. Eugene now lived in a high-rise in the financial district downtown. I didn't know what to expect when I arrived. Martin said he would be there, and so would some other family members, but we would close the door and have privacy. A man met me at the door who introduced himself as Eugene's brother-in-law. And then I met Martin, who ushered me straight into Eugene's room. He was in a hospital bed, sitting up straight, looking very alert and familiar. He couldn't offer his hand to shake because he was essentially immobilized below the neck. Apparently, he had a limited amount of motion in his left arm and leg but not much. I felt a wave of familiar joy seeing him. He was very happy to see me and completely compos mentis. Martin asked if I needed anything, brought me water, and then left us alone.

Eugene told me that he had been diagnosed almost a year ago. He moved into this apartment in January. He previously lived upstairs in a fancier place but was able to sell it for a good price and rent this one, thereby acquiring cash to distribute to his daughters. I started out by getting undressed and uncovering him. He said he would have a massage regularly in the context of occupational therapy, but he hadn't had any sensual attention since all this started. I could see that there was no point in getting fancy about full-body massage, rolling him over on his side to reach all the muscle groups. I just kissed him lightly all over, from head to toe. Then I crawled up onto the bed and made out with him, held him, touched him all over, and pleasured his penis. We reminisced about fun times we'd had in the past. He mentioned how much he enjoyed rimming, so I perched over him so he could revisit that flavor of delectation.

This was like a scene out of *The Sessions*—how does a man who can only move his tongue eat ass? That went on for only a minute—box checked. I made sure to touch him all over his body, but I assumed that primarily he wanted attention to his dick, and ultimately he admitted he wanted me to make him squirt. I manipulated him at length and then started playing with his butt, which I knew he enjoyed. I got out my Liquid Silk, slid a lubricated finger inside him, and worked his prostate while stroking him. Finally, he did yield a thick, juicy load. He asked me if it was big, and I told him; later, I realized I could have taken a picture and showed it to him. I cleaned him up. We chatted some more, and then I left. There were two women in the kitchen, presumably his caretaker and his sister, who looked at me disapprovingly. Martin walked me to the door and handed me $300, and that was that.

What struck me was how alive and alert and accepting of

his condition Eugene seemed. He told me two close friends recently visited and brought him take-out from Jean-Georges and a good bottle of Chateau Margaux. Eugene said it was everything he wanted...except one thing. The guys said, "Well, we could send you up a couple of girls from Asian Beauties." How little they knew.

Two weeks later he was gone.

CHAPTER 5

JAMES SPANKING NEW

Natasha Strange

"Natasha! Your client is here!"
This voice is definitely not part of the storyline in my book and snaps me back into reality. I've been reading in my lingerie while waiting in the changing room so all I have to do it touch up my lip gloss and slip on my heels before heading to meet...looks at appointment sheet...James Spanking New.

It's the fall of 1996. The morning air is crispy and the chill hints at this being one of the first days without the sun beating down on us by noon. Despite the chill, the man I find in the waiting room has beads of sweat on his forehead. He's slim, older, has well-trimmed graying hair. He's dressed nicely, but not in your typical Silicon Valley Dude Bro suit. More like an artist who's trying to look as if he's dressed like Dude Bro. Dude Bro cosplay. This endears him to me immediately.

"Hi James! Nice to meet you! I'm Natasha. You ready? Follow me!" I can tell he's nervous, so I try to be friendly and flirty. This usually puts a horny submissive at ease.

He doesn't move for a moment as his eyes dart to the door, then back to me, then the door...before he slowly stands and starts to follow me. I can tell he's still thinking about the door. I shimmy my ass a bit to try to distract him as I walk towards our play room in another failed attempt to distract him from the door and freedom.

He follows slowly, gripping his release form so tightly that when he hands it to me it's crumpled and sweat stained, despite him only having custody of it for a few short minutes.

I walk into our room, and point to the little bed in the corner. "Go have a seat." He pauses, then scurries past me to sit on the edge of the bed. He looks like a tiny terrified bunny. Shaking.

Perching on a chair next to the bed, I lean over and ask him how he's doing as I try to straighten the release form. I wanted to hug him and tell him it was okay.

"Fine. Fine. I'm doing fine." He shoves $120 in damp bills at me. They look to have been neatly folded in the recent past, but after spending time in his front shirt pocket have been steamed into a clump.

"Thank you. But let's talk a minute before we begin. You are interested in spanking?"

"Yes. Yes. Um. Maybe this wasn't a good idea. I don't know what I'm doing here. But...yes. Span...no. Maybe I should leave. You can just keep the money."

As nervous as he is, I expect him to say spanking AND...I don't know. Something more perverted? Something illegal? But nope. He's just terrified of spanking, despite waking up that morning, calling our number, booking the appointment, confirming from the pay phone down the street, then driving up and knocking on our door. At any of these points he could have changed his mind. Cancelled. Turned back. But he's pushing through despite being, with every fiber of his being, terrified.

"It's okay James. Spanking is not a big deal. Lots of people are interested in spanking!" I try to make light of it. To let him know I'm accepting and open and even eager to spank him.

This seems to backfire.

"No. No. I mean. I know people are into this. It's just. I've never done this before. I've never talked to anyone about this. I...no one...what would people I work with...if they knew... No. I don't know."

His breathing is coming faster and he takes his jacket off in an attempt to cool down. His thin white button-down is wet from his armpits to nearly the top of his jeans. That's the thing about kinks, non-standard sexual interests, and even being queer. Even when we know it's okay, and we are accepting of other people having those interests, it can be very difficult to admit to having those interests ourselves.

Those are great activities. For other people.

And especially in 1996 before the internet let us know that if it exists, there is porn for it.

"We don't have to do anything. We can just talk about spanking. I mean. You are here. I know that means you are curious. Do you want to hear about my last spanking session?"

This idea seems to calm him. I tell him stories about the different types of spankings I've given. The role-plays, the naughty boys who need to be punished. The implements: paddles, hair brushes, wooden spoons. That, occasionally, I switch with people I like and we take turns spanking each other.

That last bit of information makes him adjust in his seat. I can see his eyes widen, but he's still not able to make eye contact.

"I don't think I could ever spank someone."

"But do you think about it?"

"...Sometimes. But mainly I think about women spanking me."

"Our time is almost up. Do you want me to spank you just a bit? So you can feel it? You could at least lie across my lap for a bit as we talk."

"..Yes. I think that would be okay. Just with your hand."

"Sure. I'll be gentle." I say with a flirty smile. It doesn't matter. He's still not looking at me. "Can you take your pants off?"

"No! No. I'm sorry. I'm not ready for that. Can you just spank me through my jeans?"

"Of course!" I sit on the bed next to him and guide his body over my lap. I expect to feel his erection digging into my leg, but he's still far too nervous even for a fear boner.

He settles over my lap and I look down to see a wallet bulging in his back pocket.

"Can we take your wallet out of your pocket?"

"Oh god. Yes. I'm sorry." He jumps to his feet and pulls out a wallet, thick with business cards and random papers, and tosses it on the bedside table where it fluffs open like an old paperback. Then he settles over my lap a little more quickly.

I lay my hand on his butt, rubbing and patting it. I did a few light smacks while continuing our conversation. He started to open up. To talk about how he had been interested in being spanked by a woman since he was a teen. He was in his forties when I met him. The spanking itself was short, sweet and didn't even begin to redden his bottom, a feeling I knew he would grow to enjoy very much in the months and years to come.

He left the room lighter. Grinning. Holding his wallet as he didn't seem to have the mental clarity to Tetris it back into his back pocket. He had done it. He had survived his first spanking.

He had lived his first truth. Over the years I learned more about him. He was a creative. He'd won several big national awards. People in the vanilla world respect his opinion and hire him to talk in front of large audiences. Sometimes they flew him across the country to do so. He thrived in a competitive creative world in a professional capacity. But still. A little part of him always felt broken.

We often talked about how there was a Before, and an After. About how heavy that secret was to carry. How he didn't know why he didn't start exploring earlier. How the pressure to be "normal" in the bedroom had probably contributed to the demise of several of the short-lived relationships in his past. About all the spanking opportunities he had missed. About how he felt more self-confident now even when he didn't talk to anyone but me about his spanking fetish.

I worried that our sessions ended up being too much processing and not enough escapism as he started to book with pretty much everyone in the fetish house. He would check in with me frequently even as he explored with others. And looking back, that's what he needed. To explore. He had stayed hidden within himself for far too long.

I even heard that, eventually, he was able to spank a pretty girl.

CHAPTER 6

THE CASE OF SOPHIA D.

Mehdi

Sitting on the edge of the massage table Sophia asked me to rest my hands on her shoulders and head. We were in our fourth session and she had requested bodywork. As I offered the exact touch she was asking for, slowly enough to make sure I was following her specific instructions, she guided my touch with increasing confidence.

"Grab my hair, squeeze it," she commanded.

As I reached for her hair, she suddenly looked at me in a way I hadn't seen before. We had been working together for weeks now. I knew a lot about Sophia. About how her parents ignored her, how her father started having an affair when she was eight, how she had been depressed since her daughter was born seven years ago, how sex had been painful for her and how she had always felt she was too much for people.

"I was raped, anally," she said, her gaze falling. "I don't really remember much of it. I was only 16. And I was super high. I don't even know what they gave me. I was totally out of it. I knew these guys. They were friends. I know that sounds weird. What kind of friends would do that? Later, in college, I learned about rape drugs and I realized that happened to me. And then I stopped thinking about it. For a long time because I was too

ashamed. But now, right now, choosing to do this feels good."
She looked at me with a slight smile and her tone changed.

"Grab my wrists please," she requested.

As I took her wrists in my hands, I asked, "Do you feel a part of you that wants to resist this?"

"Yes. There's an angry energy rising inside me. If you were in front of me I would want to punch you." I held a cushion in front of me and gave her the option to punch hard and make any sounds she needed to. She tried punching a few times, lethargically at first and then more forcefully.

Most people are used to allowing others, especially their intimate partners (and sometimes professionals), access to their bodies without much guidance. Few get asked or get to practice asking for what they want. Trauma takes away the voice and the confidence to ask for what is truly desired. It is crucial to cultivate an attuned connection between the client and their body and a safe and consistent connection between the client and practitioner so the desires are recognized, articulated and responded to as accurately as possible. The client then feels free to explore and follow the sensations and desires as they arise to wherever they might go and to ask for appropriate responses from the practitioner. Through my training in sexological bodywork and somatic sex education and my many years working as a psychotherapist specializing in trauma and sexuality, I have developed a practice of helping people connect with their authentic selves and pleasure.

In our work together, I encouraged Sophia to trust her own intuition rather than my perceived expertise: "I don't know your body and I can't claim that you will enjoy my touch."

"Okay. Can you place your hands here...a bit firmer..." She

asked me to rest one hand in the middle of her chest and one on her belly. She directed me to press on her hips from both sides. "Touch my feet please... Yes, like that..." I felt her body relaxing under my touch. "Now walk your hands up my legs, yes slowly... Okay, stop there for a moment," she guided me with her voice. "Just gently cover my vulva... Yes, just hold me."

Sophia was testing the trust in our relationship to see who was in control and if her boundary was being respected. The more I listened to her and did precisely what she asked for, the safer she felt and the stronger her trust was in her own voice.

In the conversation afterwards, Sophia described the deep desire to communicate to her partner what would be satisfying to her erotically and how she had "gone along" in the past with what others wanted from her.

For many people, it is not clear what they want. And if they do know what they want, they might think it is too much to ask. Many questions may come up: Am I doing this right? Do I have the right to ask for this? Am I going to be rejected? Am I being selfish? If I do ask, what will be the answer?

In the following session Sophia mentioned that soon after our last session she felt suddenly confident to say no to something she had felt she had to go along with.

She spoke of her experience of giving birth to her daughter, a very long and painful labor which ended up in a hospital intervention complete with numbness under epidural, and a severe tear in her perineum about which the doctors did not tell her. There were stark similarities between this and her rape: numbness, loss of control, inability to ask for what she wanted, anal trauma, and the silence around what had in fact occurred. Was it possible that she fell into depression afterwards because the hospital experience evoked the frozen memory of the rape?

She said she had always had difficulty finding pleasure in her anal region and felt ashamed of that part of her body, even more so after the birth of her daughter. Furthermore, she felt pain in that area during sex, possibly due to scar tissues formed as a result of severe tearing.

In one session, she wanted to address the pain and the shame. She began as before by asking for various touches on different parts of her body. While she spoke her thoughts and feelings about the young man who had led the group assault, I also inquired about her body sensations. By staying attentive to both her body and her mental process, she felt different levels of release. She wanted me to put my hand around her throat as if to choke her. That was something that she typically enjoyed during sex. But in this instance, she wanted to feel the trust between us, to know I was not going to hurt her. Her intentional choice to slowly go to the edge of a danger zone allowed her to feel her sense of agency in choosing what she wanted and how she wanted to experience it. This was a deep insight: to know that she could trust someone not to push it too far and intentionally hurt her and to listen to her when she said that was enough. And even a more profound knowing—she could trust her own choice.

The challenge now was to find the edges of her boundary so that she would not have to wait until it was too late. She wanted to be able to recognize the signs along the way to know before it got to be too much. As a teenager, she was made helpless, then overpowered and violated. She had lost her ability to see the signs for what they were and the agency to direct her experience at 16. At my suggestion, she agreed to invite the presence of her teen self into the session so she could observe and learn from her mature and wise adult self.

She sat up again on the edge of the massage table and asked me to stand behind her and caress her breasts in a very specific way. "This is incredible that I can give this much direction," she said, laughing.

She instructed me to touch her upper back, then hold her around the waist. "This feels so safe." And then to hold her a bit lower, around the hips: "This feels less safe...like an alarm going off..." As she continued to guide my touch, she felt strong emotion rising inside her. She felt powerful for the first time. She felt the presence of her young teen self who wanted to be approached with care and respect.

As she asked me to slowly brush my hand on her labia, she noticed a sensation in her back that felt like the beginnings of a dissociation. She gradually verbalized how she wanted both her body to be appreciated by her lover and to do so on her own terms. But she was worried that if it became about her she would be perceived as selfish and heartless.

She lay back on the table and directed me to use warm oil to touch her vulva with my gloved hand: "Longer strokes...circle around again...more pressure on the left side..." She felt almost tearful for being able to receive what she truly wanted.

She then spoke about how her left knee hurts every time she splays her legs during sex, although that was something she loved to do. "I wonder if this knee has something to say?" I asked. Her eyes narrowed as if focusing on something or someone at a distance. She remembered a face, "This older guy, maybe 25," who bought the teens beer and was hitting on her. He got angry when she rejected him. He was probably the one who drugged her. She felt an urge to kick. Maybe kick him? I supported her knee and leg while she kicked that imaginary face.

She then asked me to keep one hand on her clitoris and slide the other under her butt cheek. This seemed to bring up a memory. With increasing anger she spoke about the boys who had disrespected her body. "If only they had taken the time to know what I wanted...maybe I would have fucked them... I would undress in front of them... I would want them to see my pussy... I'd show them my ass... But they can't fucking touch a thing... I would want them to speak to me with humility and respect...to worship me." She asked me to place my hand over her introitus, "to worship this sacred place."

Sophia was feeling her absolute power over her body and demanding respect for it. She was rewriting the assault as a sacred story of a powerful goddess. This was a work of her creative imagination. She could tune in to her own desire and ask me for a response. The unconditional meeting of her requests enabled her to grasp that deep sense of agency that had gone to sleep in her long ago. The non-prescriptive touch gave her a chance to slowly, methodically and, most importantly, in a container of pleasure and relational safety, find and release the traumatic experiences that were held in different parts of her body.

Sophia and I had a total of seven 90-minute sessions. In a follow-up interview a few months later she shared, "There has been a significant shift in my stress tolerance. I feel now more able to ask my partner specifically for what I want without demanding but also with a sense of patience and understanding if it doesn't go my way. What's been most meaningful is in my interactions around sex and intimacy overall: I am experiencing nothing short of a revolution in my standards being raised for what I will put up with and how I ask for my needs, emotional and physical, to be met."

CHAPTER 7

FOUR DAYS

Daddy Lance

It's the summer of 2014 and I'm in my Chrysler Crossfire winding through the sharp curves of the 101 along the coast of Northern California. I left San Francisco three and a half hours ago and I am ready to finish my trip, stretch my legs and meet the incredible man I have been talking to for the last month and a half. I'm now only about 20 minutes from Fort Bragg, a town on the Mendocino coast known for its beach that is dotted with colorful glass stones. I see the driveway ahead. I make a left turn and see that it splits ahead of me, each leading to separate properties with large houses by the ocean. I bear to the right and toward the beige house. The design isn't my taste, but the location is everything. I park my car in front of the house and start taking out my luggage. It's only a four-day trip, but I've packed as if I'm going to be there for over a week. Despite all our discussions leading up to this day, I'm still uncertain as to what we might all get up to, so I've overpacked out of an abundance of caution. We are at least three hours from an "adult novelty" shop, so if suddenly he wanted to try nipple clamps and I hadn't brought any, we'd be screwed.

As I approach the door it slowly opens before I've even had a chance to knock. He had likely been waiting at the door for a while, eagerly anticipating my arrival. As the door opens, I finally lay my eyes on John, and he seems incredibly happy and excited. I step inside and quickly put my bags down as I can feel just how much he needs me to wrap my arms around him. I kneel down and do just that, squeezing and pulling him slightly away from the wheelchair that he requires for mobility. John has a condition which is causing his muscles to atrophy over time. For now, he is able to stand up, but does not have enough strength to walk. He's been in a wheelchair for about five years.

John reached out to me through my website after an exhaustive search for someone who could help him "learn what it means to be a gay man." John had been married until a year and a half ago when his wife passed away. He was aware of his same-sex attraction from a very early age, but coming out in the 1950s never seemed an option. He did as he was supposed to, got married (though never had kids) and became very successful. He had worked as an executive for a large, international engineering firm and retired well. He loved his wife dearly and had no regrets about the choice he made to spend most of his life with her. From that deep love he never explored his same-sex attraction in physical form.

He shared with me that he had been looking at ads and websites of probably a hundred different men over the last six months, trying to find the person with the experience, compassion and patience to take him on this journey of exploration and education. He also stated that it didn't hurt he found me incredibly attractive and loved that I'm well endowed. Over the next six weeks we exchanged dozens of emails, which often were more like short stories. I could tell he could write, and write well. A simple inventory of what he had in the kitchen and what he planned to pick up before I arrived flowed like poetry. He let me know all of the sexual things he hoped to explore, that he definitely wanted to have oral sex and also really wanted to get fucked. He had already purchased a sling online, which has been sitting in his garage, unopened. He also stated that he'd got some dildos that he'd been playing with and had learned about douching. I was impressed by the things he shared with me. He had taken a proactive step toward self-pleasure and preparation even before I arrived. Still, I am not sure how quickly we'll get to full, penetrative anal sex, but I figure over the course of our four days together, anything is possible.

As I hug him, I can feel his heart against mine, I can hear how quickly it's beating, I can feel his mix of anxiety and excitement. I can feel how deeply he has needed this, not just in this moment, but his entire life, a deep, connected, intimate hug. The hug lasts maybe a minute. I'm not going to pull away until he is ready. I finally feel him completely relax and I slowly release. Cradling his face in my hands I look into his eyes for a moment and then give him his "first" kiss.

He compliments me on my little sports car and asks how the drive was as he shows me to the bedroom where I drop off my bags. He gives me a little tour around the house. It has a theatre room, which gets me starting to think about what essential gay movies we should watch. He also shows me into the garage, where sure enough, there is the sling, still in its discreet packaging. He also shows me the large accessible van that I will be driving us around in over the next few days.

We make our way back to the living room and he asks if I'd like some wine. He pours us both a glass, and sits down next to me. We had covered so much in our emails that we don't need to start with basic background questions, so he shares the more intimate details of how long he'd been married, when they met, and how he knows that she would be happy for him right now, as he's being authentic to himself. As he speaks, I caress his knee for a while, then his inner thigh. He places his hand on top of mine and I can feel gentleness in his touch. I wrap one arm around him, pulling him in even closer to me and he happily nuzzles into my chest. After maybe 30 minutes, as I finish my glass of wine, he says, "Can we get naked now?" "Absolutely!" I reply. "Can we set up the sling first?" he asks. I'm a little surprised that he is bringing up the sling so soon. "Sure," I reply, "there's plenty of room and we will get there eventually."

We walk into the bedroom and he locks his wheelchair in place and stands up in front of me. I wrap my arms around him cradling and supporting him, taking some deep breaths and connecting to each other's energy. I then undress myself before helping him to undress. Though I know he is perfectly capable of undressing himself, there is something wonderfully intimate about allowing someone to undress you, and I want to share that intimacy with him. Once we are both naked, I pull him once more for another hug, though of course a more intimate one as our bare chests, stomachs and cocks touch. When we pull away, we are both visibly aroused and I invite him to touch my cock if he likes. He doesn't hesitate in accepting my invitation. He says he thinks he should freshen up a little bit, and wheels himself into the bathroom. While he is in the bathroom, I grab the sling from the garage and bring it into the bedroom, where I began setting it up in the corner of the large room. It's a little different from the one I have at home, aluminum versus steel, but the general engineering is the same, so I get it assembled within a few minutes. Once done, I climb into bed and wait for him to arrive from the bathroom. He's taking a while in the bathroom, which I assume means he is douching.

If you're not a person who participates in passive anal sex or someone who enjoys the benefits of colonic irrigation then you don't know how complex and time consuming douching can be. It also can become a source of anxiety for many, making sure that they are entirely cleaned out, with no excess water. I have had many clients share stories of being shamed for not being perfectly clean when they bottomed, some even by other "professionals" (if you can't handle it, this probably isn't the right job for you). Because of this, I try to exhibit plenty of patience, though I certainly feel bad when it takes a client 30 minutes of his one-hour session just to "get ready."

John finally emerges from the bathroom, rolls over to the bed and climbs in to join me. Lying on our sides, facing one another, I pull him in to me, resting his head on my chest, his body lightly trembles with excitement. Once I feel his body relaxing a bit I release my firm hold, pull away and we begin to kiss. As we begin to kiss more deeply and passionately, my cock responds quite positively and he can feel me growing hard against his leg. He reaches down and wraps his hand around my cock, which brings a huge smile to his face. He asks if he can suck it, to which I respond, "Yes, please." I slide up on the bed a little bit while he slides down and he begins to worship my dick with his mouth and hands. He's very attentive and concerned about "doing things right" and I assure him it feels wonderful. I give him a little feedback about the differences between pleasuring an uncut cock (which I have) versus a cut one, in terms of how the sensitivity of the head is different. He thanks me for the information and returns to my cock, paying special attention to the foreskin and all the wonderful nerves it contains.

After maybe five minutes I usher him back up to me where we begin kissing again. I can now feel his cock pressing hard against my stomach. I rotate him on his side and then on his back and take my turn, moving down the bed to suck his cock. The moment my tongue touches the sensitive head of his cut cock he lets out a deep moan of ecstasy. As I pleasure and worship his cock, he continues to affirm how amazing it feels, that he never knew it could feel so good. I can feel his cock pulsing hard and I want to make sure that I don't take him to orgasm too quickly, so I slow things down a bit, lightly caressing his inner thighs and stomach, moving the energy around. After another few minutes I return to kissing and cuddling him.

As we hold one another I slide my hand down his back to the crack of his ass and begin to lightly stroke his hole. I reach behind me, grab the bottle of lube off of the bedside table, squirt a little in my hand and return to his hole, slightly penetrating him with my lubed-up finger. He begins to moan ecstatically again and I can feel him slightly pushing his ass toward my finger, asking for more. He opens up more, so I insert a second finger and then a third. We return to deep, passionate kissing as I gently make love to his hole with my three fingers. After several minutes of this he asks if we can move to the sling. I'm surprised that he's asking to get in the sling (presumably to get fucked) quite so soon, but I figure if he is ready, so am I. After all, he's waited 60 years for this. Who am I to say it's too soon?

He scoots to the edge of the bed and I help him stand up.

He grabs the frame of the sling for support, takes a few steps around and, with my help, drops into the sling. I put his legs into the stirrups and then check in to make sure he's comfortable. He assures me he is very comfortable and I return my attention to his ass, fingering him while I rub his head and we make out. Once I can feel that he can comfortably handle three of my fingers, I make my way around to the end of the sling and between his legs. I lube up my cock and then check in with him, asking if he is ready for it. He says he is and I promise that I will take my time. I penetrate him with just the head and I can feel him tighten a bit (the first few inches are sometimes the toughest). I pull out for a minute and encourage him to take a couple deep breaths. Once I can feel him relax a bit I penetrate him again and can feel he isn't tightening as much. I leave my dick just a few inches inside him and encourage him to continue deep breathing, while making sure I am listening to my own body. As I feel him open a bit more, I slowly push deeper and deeper until I am fully inside him.

His eyes grow wild. He is speechless and clearly thrilled. While staying inside him, I lean down on him and kiss him deeply, then wrap my arms under the sling and around him. I can feel his heart pounding under mine. He moans into my ear and says, "I can't believe this is happening. You feel amazing!" I continue to fuck him for probably ten minutes until I can tell that he's starting to feel a bit worn out. Leaving my dick inside him, I stop thrusting, just leaving it in place while I move the energy we've created through the rest of his body, caressing his legs, from inner thigh to the tips of his toes, then his tummy, chest, shoulders and arms to the tip of his fingers. My cock begins to soften until I finally fall out of him. I lean down once again and wrap my arms around him and ask how he's doing. "Amazing," he replies, "I never knew it could feel so good! You are so wonderful and caring." I almost begin to cry as I can feel how his words are truly coming from his soul and what a profound moment this is for him, something he has only been able to fantasize about for so long. We return to the bed and the play and cuddling lasts for another hour, until it is dinner time.

The next three days were filled with wonderful conversations at his home and on the road as he showed me around the North Central coast. He told me stories of all the adventures and travels he experienced through his work and alongside his wife. He shared with me moments when he had opportunities to act on his same-sex attraction and didn't. For example, when he was in early high school and a boy caught him "looking" while they were both at the urinal. The boy grabbed him, pushed him into a stall, closed the door and demanded that he suck his cock. Though a part of him was intrigued, the aggression of the situation made him retreat. On another occasion he was in the Middle East, waiting for his taxi to arrive, when a limo pulled up. After a few moments the driver exited, approached him and informed him that his boss would like to spend some time with him and would make it worth it for him. Again, his fear superseded his intrigue and he declined the request.

As planned, we watched some gay movies, including my favorite, *Sordid Lives*, with the late Leslie Jordan. He told me he hoped to find someone, younger but not too young, who could be a friend, lover and caregiver. Someone who would live with him, share laughs, love and also be able to help care for him.

In exchange, he would leave them his estate. If I didn't already have a boyfriend (who is now my husband) I would have given the idea great consideration.

The morning of the fourth day came more quickly than I expected. As I packed my bags, I felt an abundance of gratitude that I got to share this experience with him. As we said our goodbyes, he said that he felt like a completely different man to the man he'd been before I arrived and that he would never forget our time and hoped we could connect again down the road.

Over the next few months we shared a few emails and he let me know that he had been chatting with a young man who was planning to come visit him toward the end of the year. It was about another year when I got an email saying that the guy had come down for Christmas and never left, and just a few months ago, they had a small marriage ceremony surrounded by a few close friends. Though I was a bit sad that this likely meant we would never meet again, I was happy that he had found companionship and hopefully the next great love of his life.

In preparation for writing this I decided to do an online search for his name. I was saddened to find his obituary from a year and a half ago. This referenced his late wife and parents, his surviving siblings and extended family, his passion for music, and finally, in reference to his husband, "will be missed by... his friend and caregiver."

I am struck by the wording but not surprised. I know his friend and caregiver was much more than that. The important thing is they had those years together. Just as we had our four days together. John had learned exactly what it was to be a gay man.

CHAPTER 8

SEX GOD

Eva Alio

"I want to be a sex god."

—M

M was taller than me and very attractive. In his early thirties, he had been avoiding penetrative sex as much as possible for over ten years. He described himself as having erectile dysfunction, premature ejaculation and past sexual trauma. He was surrounded by porn culture and had huge performance anxiety. This aspect of his life was secret and in direct opposition to his very public and very popular persona of being a dominant, sexual virtuoso.

M's goal was to gain more understanding about penetrative sex so he could feel confident in navigating his sexual relationships moving forward. He wanted to have penetrative sex with his new partner and was tired of being afraid. He had explored his sexuality with partners in all areas except this. M had booked a three-day intensive and was here with me, dropping his ego and farce in order to face his fear of penetration and sexual failure head on.

M was good at expressing himself: telling me how he was feeling, what he was feeling, how he was doing. He said he was not this way with everyone in his life, or even in his intimate but platonic relationships. He recognized that he had a perspective of viewing sex and emotional intimacy as two different, irreconcilable things. He wanted to know if he could bring the two together: penetrative sex and intimacy. I normalized this because it is not uncommon. Reconciling these two things has also been my path. It was a privilege to be around M this way. I love to be real. I loved his realness.

I met him outside and we chatted at the park first. The walk and weather were good for releasing excess nervousness. When we got cold, we headed back to the house. At home, we wrapped up the introductory talk and then, gauging his comfort level, I asked him if he ever just hung out naked.

I said, "It's great for normalizing nudity. What would you think if we did the rest of the session without clothes on, and just let our inner children be innocent, playful and curious?"

He was dubious but totally game.

We undressed. I invited him to look at me and slowly turned in a circle. Then he did the same.

After that, I invited him into the mirror talk. Again, dubious but game. Mirror talk is where one person looks in the mirror and talks about the form, function and their feelings about their body. The other person remains silent, to observe and witness. I went first, talking about what I loved and didn't love about my body. The struggles I've had being in it. Pointing and touching different parts. When I was done, I felt a bit shaky with the vulnerability and exposure. He reflected understanding, appreciation and awe of my vulnerability and was hesitant to go next. He didn't have to and he knew that. I watched him make the choice. He looked in the mirror and talked about his insecurities and difficulties. The things he struggled with and the things he liked. After that we breathed together again, into our bellies, making eye contact a bit until things settled. Then I invited him to sit on the couch.

We paused, turned the lights down and softened into the couches, allowing our bodies to make consensual contact. I gently told him we were not there to practice tolerating things. We were not there to practice discomfort.

There was a natural progression into a hand caress. I got some baby powder and invited him to give me his arm, to allow me to find my pleasure in touching it. His job was simply to feel where my skin touched his and notice the sensations in his body from it. He did. It was heavenly. He said, "Why doesn't everyone do this? Know this?" Exactly. Then he touched my arm. He was surprised at how intimate it was, at how close and connected he felt to me. Then we did the other arm, and when it was his turn again, he requested both of my arms. The presence and beauty were so palpable by the end I had tears running down my face. I said, "This is sex, too."

.M's self-awareness and ability to ride his own edge was powerful. He was aware when he was losing presence and capable of grounding himself back into it.

Beautiful Being, THESE are the skills of the sex god. Pure, authentic presence. When you have that, you naturally develop attunement to your partner. It's exquisite.

Before the end of the session, I invited him into a genital tour, me showing mine and naming parts, him showing his. Afterwards, M said his inner child felt like a little buddha, so very calm. He said he was a convert to nakedness and playfully complained about having to put his clothes back on. We ended the session with a gentle kiss—a closing of this day and a beckoning bud of beauty to come back with tomorrow.

DAY 2

We started naked on the bed, catching up about our days, doing body scans to feel the feelings and anxieties. M said he had the urge to have alcohol and I normalized that, then told him a funny story from my day and we laughed about the absurdity of malfunctioning smoke alarms. We continued to intentionally relax and soften into our bodies.

We reviewed Betty Martin's wheel of consent. I presented my proposal for the evening: We could play and explore, allowing the sexual energy to rise, and if he felt inclined, he could initiate condom placement at any time. We didn't have to do anything with or about it. We could use as many condoms as we felt like. Also, he could initiate/ask for penetration. I wouldn't initiate. His ingrained experience was of women wanting penetration and him avoiding it. We would have no expectations other than to feel our bodies and be in the present moment.

Then we talked through what might happen and the course of action forward: Condom on and goes soft? Smile, stay in our senses, put all attention on the touch and feeling happening. Relax and enjoy. Penetration and goes soft? We stay connected, not moving, and bring awareness to the feeling of our bodies, bring awareness to the connection, breathe, soften and allow the energy of our closeness to flow. We follow the pleasure of our closeness and connection.

Penetration and rapid ejaculation? Enjoy the ejaculation! Allow the pleasure of it. Accept it. We talked about the moment of ejaculation inevitability and the body sensations that happen before that, noticing that if we are being present and mindful, he would be able to feel these things happening. He would be aware. This made sense to him. I also talked about emotional bursts of energy and allowing space for those to move or sound. I said if he felt fear or like running away, that was his cue to slow down. In direct opposition to his normal pattern, I invited him in those moments to get closer to me, to slow down and lean into my presence and love, lean into my acceptance and the truth of the moment. M took a long breath but nodded solemnly. We were on the same page.

I asked if I could find pleasure by caressing his body. I used baby powder and my body to slide, glide and feel. He requested a condom. After a time, he asked me to get on top and we had nice, penetrative sex. Then M got quieter and quieter. I asked if I could slide off and just caress his whole body again. Yes. I did. I asked where it would feel most delicious. His cock. M softened, breathed and relaxed into his body, feeling and naming the sensations. I caressed and feather danced my fingers on his cock, naming sensations. I said it felt like playing an instrument. He said it was as if his cock was making the sound of the gentle music emanating from the speaker. I said, "Is that why it's called a skin flute?" We both laughed. Laughter is good in bed.

Raspberry noises on our sweaty bodies made me laugh, as well as trying not to fart.

M shared about what he had just experienced. When he felt his sexuality rising and he wanted to penetrate, what he calls *unleashing his wild side*, is when he clamped down and feared performance failure, that was why he had gone quiet.

He wanted to engage more and then shut it down. I tried to describe being in your body and attuned for the escalation of excitement, too, but these things are hard, if not impossible, to learn by words alone.

Time was running low and we talked more about his desire for unleashing. I restated that anxiety and fear are cues to slow down and get really present with the feeling happening, and if available, to lean into me. Feel the fear and bring it into the space between us. He wanted to try, so we agreed to experiment even though there was only 15 minutes left on the time. I roused my own body into excitement and receptivity by feeling into his masculine drive and desire. "What do you feel inside?" I asked. M stood still with his eyes closed, feeling into his sexuality, and said, "I want to be a little bit aggressive." "What would that look like?" I said slowly. "Will you show me?" He breathed, his body's energy cupping around mine, and placed a hand on my throat. We played with this a few times and my body responded with receptivity and arousal, as did his. "Will you put a condom on?" he asked. I did. I am best at this skill with my mouth, so that is how I prefer to do it. I whispered, "What wants to come out of you now? Will you show me?" He asked me to turn around. I invited him to take action on his urge. He did. Entering, thrusting and experiencing, then turning me around and thrusting some more. This let off after only a minute and we regrouped and debriefed a bit. He was jubilant at the experience. Now we knew where the playing field was for the next day.

DAY 3

We looked at each other. A long look. The presence was ripe.

M had come to the crux of what he showed up to work on—having penetrative sex while maintaining connection and intimacy. It is rare for a client to move as quickly as he did. M had been in therapy for years and had a firm understanding of his body and his window of tolerance for self-regulating. He had explored his sexuality alone with himself and with partners but with very little penetration for years. With me, he had been regulating, absorbing and integrating our work together at a phenomenal rate, then asking for more. I had been at his side, watching, guiding and inviting. It was because of M's already developed ability to be present, intimate, attuned and self-aware that we were able to explore and experience his sexuality at such depth and in such a short amount of time.

We were naked and gave each other a hug of gratitude and acknowledgement. It didn't end. I felt the beauty and the raw power in him that were longing to be out. Longing to be free. My body responded. I told him he was powerful. His sexual energy was powerful. His cock was powerful, no matter how it showed up. Did he feel me? Yes. Picking up from the previous day I ask again, "What is your expression now? Will you show me?" And he did, the hand lightly caressing my throat, the breath coming harder. My body melted under his. A doorway of possibilities opened.

I kept drawing his power out with my own. "Show me," I whispered. He groaned and asked for a condom. Mindfully and slowly, I obliged.

Then we were fucking again but this time he was more centered. He was more in himself and he became more and more centered the more he relaxed into what was happening and what he was feeling. He was feeling his cock and he was feeling me. My body was feeling him. My body felt safe and connected with the presence he was bringing. The sweet spot at my cervix opened a little. The more conscious he was, the more receptive my body was.

He was aware, connected to me, in his body, and we were in it together. I slid back on the bed and we were drenched in sweat. He was present and eager. He asked if I would ride him and I did, not keeping a steady rhythm but rather following the rhythm of our bodies. Feeling. The connection deepened. I rode and modulated with his energy, slowing down and picking up as nature moved through us.

At slower times we spoke out loud the sensations in our bodies. I said, "I feel your hands on my hips, the sweat where my skin touches yours, warmth in my belly and expansion in my heart." He said, "I feel the heat of you surrounding my cock. I hear my own breathing, the music and feel the sheets bunching at my feet. Your skin is so soft." In this presence, I was awash in extended moments of ethereal levitation. I leaned all the way forward, chest to chest, my cheek next to his. We were not moving forward but suspended, blossoming. M breathed into my ear, "This is what sex is for, isn't it?..." "Yes" is all I could murmur, getting even closer. Time slowed. Intimacy expanded. Pleasure widened. My invisible body softened more, encompassing his. I whispered that I felt like stardust dancing in the milky way. I drew him into me even as he drew me into him.

The chair that was acting as a headboard for my air mattress slid away from the bed and M's head fell into the crevasse. I laughed and pulled on him. "Come back this way," I said breathlessly. He scooched more onto the bed and in doing so

I found myself sitting in his lap, legs around his torso. Time swirled and distorted. This position of greatest spiritual alignment had never been so comfortable and I'd never understood what it was for. But the longer we were there, not moving except for pulses and squeezes and eye gazing, the more I felt nature's intertwining of our ethereal sparks. I felt the goddess in me expand, energy in my womb opening downward to receive from the earth and energy at the top opening to receive spirit. There in the middle, this was where we met. In our bodies. Spirit entwined in flesh and earth. I laughed. M was gazing at me. "Who are you?" he said. "What are you doing to me?" "I don't know!" I said laughing. "But I love it."

I looked at him again, and to continue our game of being present and speaking out loud I asked myself, *What am I feeling?* Then out loud I gave the answer, "No separation. I feel no separation." I laughed and felt his embrace squeezing me even closer. I felt his cock and looked into his gaze. I felt my womb space softly emanating joy all around us. I felt surrounded by love, space and stars. I felt timeless and unbound, not moving yet everything was slowly in motion.

We just stayed. It was effortless to be in this place. He appeared to be having a wondrous experience of his own. And yet, we were in it together.

We came down and disengaged slowly. "I don't want to lose the connection," he murmured when I leaned too far back and he slipped out. I scooched closer and asked if I could cuddle. We did. We merged into the space, basking in the magnetics that had been created. I felt nourished, wholesome, filled, peaceful. He wondered at the atmosphere that had been created, murmuring that he'd never felt this way before and certainly not after being sexual. I said to him, "Perhaps this is what an afterglow is."

And then with a voice he could not hear with his ears..."You are a sex god."

CHAPTER 9

RUBIX CUBE

Eva Alio

A friend of mine invited me to a Friday evening social event. She sidled up to me, singled out a friend of hers and said, "You should talk to him. He needs your coaching."

Her friend Rubix was in his early seventies, hetero, friendly and personable, and we struck up a conversation. Rubix has had a personal practice of using mantra repetition for meditation for 40 years. He'd had three marriages end and was on a mission to find spiritual, physical and sexual intimacy with a woman. When I explained intimacy and connection coaching for sex and love from the somatic viewpoint—how I help people change the conditioning in their minds and nervous systems—he exclaimed what our mutual friend had predicted, "I need your work!"

He was only in town for a week and booked my free two-hour consultation for the following Monday. The consultation went really well and he booked three more sessions in the following three days.

Newly minted in my coaching certification, I'd probably done close to 100 sessions for practice or trade. Rubix was the first person to pay me for my coaching.

The coaching methodology is effective by working with the felt sense in our bodies. We relax and become mindful to what signals our body presents when faced with the possibility of having our desires. We can emphasize these body sensations when we use a Five Senses Reality practice; envision having the desire and bring all our senses online—how does it look, touch, taste, smell, sound? At first, the client experiences success in their body/mind/emotions at having attained their goal. This in itself is hugely valuable as it signals to the body what *is* possible! Then when the client is asked to scan for any resistance, obstacles to the desire will usually object quite clearly in physical form. For example, my heart is heavy, my throat is constricted, my shoulder hurts, my belly is nauseous!

From there I have tools to guide folks into gaining clarity around the message from the nervous system. It is common for these parts to be outdated safety mechanisms, pockets of stuck energy that developed to protect our vulnerable, authentic selves. These places can get uncomfortably triggered when we go toward what we want. It can be what makes getting what we want seem anywhere from difficult to impossible. Clarity, acceptance and understanding create space and grow our awareness. Then we can take care of this part of us. From the inside out, our nervous systems unwind blockages and the outward change in our lives is natural, feels good and is not forced.

After the integration process, I guide clients in ways that will carve these new paths deeper into their physical system—with imagination, intentional breathing and solo sacred sexuality or pleasure practices. Over time, more and more of the true nature of our body-mind becomes liberated for presence, pleasure and awareness. We become more whole, more free.

It's a beautiful process. I was getting comfortable with it, gaining skill and...

None of it was working for Rubix.

The first coaching session fell flat. He would immediately sink into a spacious mind and the warm, open, loving kindness of his heart. Nothing else going on in his body. I had done exercises with him during the consult, so I knew he had body awareness. I knew he could tap into his felt sense. This was weird.

Rubix's biggest and most urgent complaint was that it was only during the previous two years he'd begun to discover how much he had lacked intimacy and deep connection in his life. He'd been on a mission, going to trainings and taking classes to try and figure it all out. He even did three weeks of workshops for sacred sexuality and spirituality in one year! He put himself in places with opportunities for intimacy, sex and exploration with willing, skilled women. He wanted it, desired it, craved it... and while his cock worked fine for him when he was alone— self-pleasure was good and he still woke up with erections during the night—it had been over four years since he'd been hard in the presence of a woman. Even with enhancements...nothing.

An erection is not an essential piece for good lovemaking, but I could see how this would be a stumper that might drive a man a bit crazy.

Rubix didn't feel anything in his body from it. Just a block in his existence that whirled and suffered and drove him to follow "the bread crumbs of truth." He could see other people having what he wanted, but for him, "it just wasn't landing."

Rubix felt our coaching session fell flat, too. He came back the next day and voiced his concerns. He wanted the embodiment—where was the embodiment I had so passionately talked about? I was aware of the stalemate.

After that first session, I pivoted. I wanted to find a way to use Rubix's success in meditation as a bridge into his body. Something he would understand intuitively and it would naturally incorporate moving forward. For his second session, I asked Rubix if he was open to doing something more ritualized, and if so, would he bring a token for his *ishta devata* (part of his meditation practice) to place on the altar? When he agreed, I went out and bought a bag of peaches and a loaf of bakery bread.

In this session, his mental block said he couldn't imagine or create an internal experience of something he'd been deprived of his whole life. This ability to create with our imagination is one of our most valuable tools as humans. We got very clear on his desire as an intention for the day: "I desire to have deeply spiritual, sensual, sexual, mutual connection and intimacy with a physical lover who accepts me and wants to be with me as much as I want to be with them."

In the ritual space, with enough relaxation, openness and experimenting, we were able to provide conditions for him to have a successful five senses reality experience. We were fully clothed and he sat across from me, breathing with his eyes closed. I guided him to welcome his dream lover. He had a full body response then. She was there. He was feeling her, seeing her, tasting, smelling and hearing her. His senses came alive. He was blown away. He came out of the experience to exclaim, "Can we do that again? Please!" We did.

Afterwards, we shared the peaches from the altar and I sent him home with the loaf of bread. On the bag I had written, "You deserve more than crumbs."

The next morning, he texted to say he felt as if "something

woke up inside him." He could put his attention on "her" and immediately he felt his senses come alive.

For our third session, I brought sensate focus tools into the ritual space. He was so anxious about performance! I gently took his hands in mine and faced him. We chatted first, about what we had for breakfast, how we liked our tea. He settled. We kept our underwear on and his task was to put all his well-cultivated meditation attention into his body sensations, to allow himself to receive touch and be aware of the felt sense of it. Sitting across from one another again, in the first minute he began to soften, leaning forward until the top of his head rested on my chest. My hands caressed with nurturing, nourishing, tender loving kindness. "I've never received touch like this from a woman before," he said. Tears rolled down my face. He softened more. Then he turned around, laid his back against my chest, and melted.

"I didn't know it was okay for me to be soft," he murmured. As my body spoke to his, the conditioning that said softness in a man is weakness began to melt away.

When he was ready to switch, I allowed him, within our agreed boundaries, to touch my body. I had explained that instead of touching me for my pleasure and trying to ask, guess or figure out what that was, he was to continue to be present in his body, in this moment only, to touch for his pleasure and to have all of his attention on his senses. We had done short practices previously that were a foundation for this and he had done plenty of such exercises in the workshops he'd attended. When I had explained the practice for today I looked him in the eyes and said I wanted to invite him into the experience of touching a woman who is soft, receptive and in her own pleasure. This way he could experience what attunement to that would be like. For his present, attuned touch, I would allow my body to soften, receive and authentically respond with breathing, sound and movement.

It was lovely. We kept a running dialogue throughout. Rubix enjoyed the fact that we could talk and bring awareness to all the felt sense happenings without dampening the sensual experience. My favorite part was his fascination with my thighs. While he was still sitting with his back against my chest, he kept strolling his fingertips along my legs as they were wrapped around his torso. He said they were so soft, like divine pillows. I laughed and squeezed him, promising my thighs I would treat them more like that in future.

Rubix booked a fourth session for the next day, the last day before leaving town. I proposed three hours and had clear direction, with a plan.

When he arrived, I drew the two triangles that made a six-pointed star, explaining each of them simply. One is active and one is receptive (traditionally called masculine and feminine); then I put a dot in the center, representing the union of opposites. I asked if he felt as if he'd been more in one triangle than the other his whole life. Yes, of course, the upward pointing triangle, the active one. But you want this dot in the middle, right? The union of opposites... Yes. Wouldn't it make sense that to be a whole human, to be this star, one would have to be familiar with both triangles? Just think! If a person did that inside themselves, if a man identified with the active principle became more familiar with the receptive principle inside himself...is it possible that a natural consequence of that work would result in the feminine outside him ceasing to become so evasive, mysterious and challenging? Rubix didn't take long to answer... Yes.

I proposed the plan. For all three hours I invited him to become the downward pointing triangle; the receptive. Let go of everything and become only the nature of his body which is made of earth, the elements, his senses, and the softness of femininity when it is loved and adored.

For the first hour I asked if he would allow and receive touch to the entirety of his naked body that was exploratory, innocent and curious. Playful even. We would "map" his body.

He would pay attention and rate the sensitivity of each place on a scale of 1 to 10. Then he would rate the sensation of the touch as nurturing, sensual or sexual.

For the next 30 minutes, using what we'd just learned, he would direct me toward how he wanted to be touched and where, for the sheer sake of the enjoyment of it.

For the last hour we would open the ritual space and he would allow me to be the active person. He would stay in his role of the receptive, receiving love, intimacy and connection to the felt sense of his body. I would bring erotic energy and attune to him but I would not touch or stimulate any part of him for the purpose of orgasm. I invited him to revel in his senses...and in this.

He agreed.

For all of this we had clear boundaries communicated, understood, agreed on and in place.

For the first hour Rubix discovered parts of his body he didn't know could be so delightfully felt and sensual. I caressed the underside of his penis, and when it was far more sensitive than stroking the top, he exclaimed, "You'd think after 70 years I would know that!" He also hadn't known how heavenly feather touches all over his whole body could be. He loved having his feet caressed.

For the 30 minutes of touching for enjoyment he chose three parts: head, feet, genitals.

For the last hour, to open the ritual space I read to him about the mystery of the primordial Goddess. Then I shed my dress and spoke my intent, looking into his eyes, "May the divine in me recognize the divine in you. May it pour into you lifetimes of love lost." He caught his breath and was so very, very moved. He kissed my forehead and murmured his intent, "To be in the flow."

Then he laid back and I allowed love to pour through me, his body and inner world receiving it like a sponge. No body fluid contact, no sexual stimulation of organs, just a deep, spiritual and sexual recognition of myself in another with skin-to-skin contact...and wouldn't you know it... He got hard.

I want to always remember the look on his face: amazement, disbelief, relief and as if he wanted to get up, shout and dance around. He laughed and called me Goddess Durga, his *ishta devata*. He pulled me close with gratitude and I received the embrace, allowing my heart to stay connected to his.

I continued to explore and play with his body, even to explore his hard cock gently and curiously with my hands, following the pleasure, reveling in it, but not chasing. Not forcing. Not expecting, wanting, anticipating or making it mean anything other than pleasure in this moment.

The energy naturally subsided. The session wrapped. We showered the coconut oil off and closed the ritual space.

I messaged Rubix the next day to check in. I celebrated how

wise I thought his penis was. I said perhaps his cock was wiser than both of us when it came to the truth about sex, connection and intimacy. I wondered if perhaps he might do very well to continue listening to and learning from his cock. I offered the suggestion and instructions for testicle massage—a technique known to increase sexual security, connection and vulnerability for penis owners.

And I encouraged him to put his attention on his internal lover when he invokes her. To shower her with love, adoration and tenderness. To learn about her, attune to her, be present with her. To use his senses every day in more ways than he ever imagined possible and to invite continual wonder at the unfolding and evolving truth of nature within us.

CHAPTER 10

WE MET AT THE MUSEUM

Wendy

When I was in my late twenties, I decided to try sex work. The inspiration came from my grandparents' friend Sheldon. Sheldon's wife of over 50 years had recently passed and he was clearly lonely. He sat at my grandparents' small dining table and talked about how he'd got "a girl." She helped prepare meals, do light cleaning, keep him company. As he was talking, I could hear the sadness in his tone. He had kids and grandkids but I'm pretty sure he only had one romantic love in his life and she was gone. I thought of what it was like for him to be in the same apartment they shared for so many years, the same bed.

It occurred to me that Sheldon could maybe use a little affection in his life. I doubted his girl was supplying that. Of course not, it wasn't her job. But I wondered if Sheldon would like a girl whose job it was. I didn't imagine he was craving sex so much as a gentle touch, someone to hold him, someone to hold. And who knows, maybe a little sexy time? And I thought, I could do that. I could be *that* girl. I certainly wasn't going to proposition Sheldon, my grandparents' longtime friend. But there must be other Sheldons out there. I was living in New York City, where anything and everything is possible.

My goal was to find one regular client, a sort of sugar daddy, to keep it simple and low risk. I was in graduate school studying sexuality and the whole idea was fascinating to me, as well as titillating. I was also low on cash. I put an ad in the *Village Voice*. This was in the before days, when personal ads were charged per word. No photos, no links, no social media. I studied the ads of others who I assumed were selling sex in the back pages of the paper, but not stating it explicitly. My final line was: "I'll spoil you, if you spoil me."

The calls started to roll in. I had very little to go on, just the sound of someone's voice. Did they seem kind? Were they taking me seriously? I began arranging meet and greets. Always in a restaurant, in a neighborhood I knew. I met many interesting men and what struck me most was what else they were looking for aside from sex. A companion, someone to listen to them, laugh at their jokes, maybe even like them. I had expected to be turned on by the idea. I was quite the exhibitionist, and the idea of sharing my body with someone in exchange for money was arousing. What I didn't expect was how much compassion I would feel for the men. They weren't pushy, the way I had seen Johns portrayed in the movies or on TV. Perhaps it was because I had chosen the ones with the kindest voices. They seemed vulnerable. They weren't interviewing me. I was interviewing them.

I also recognize my inherent privilege in this. I am white, middle class, cisgender, and at the time young, thin and more or less what one would consider conventionally attractive. Not drop dead gorgeous, more along the cute spectrum. I decided this worked in my advantage with men as I was pretty enough, but not so much as to be intimidating. If I had been anything other than these things, I could have had a very different, not so positive, experience.

Because I was new to this world and had no one to guide me, except for my therapist, who was also new to this world, I opted for the man who seemed most at home with the transactional nature of our relationship. He insisted we meet at the restaurant at the Guggenheim. He told me he only donated money there and nowhere else. As if that was something that would impress me. It was because of his generous donations that we could be dining here. He said if people asked how we met, we would say it was at the museum. He looked less like a sugar daddy and more like a sugar granddaddy. I was in my twenties and he was in his seventies. I thought people who knew me might think it odd that I was picking up old men at the museum as lunch dates, but luckily we never needed to explain our relationship to anyone.

At our lunch meeting, he slipped me an envelope that I later discovered had $100 in it.

I had not requested any payment for what I saw as his interview. I was impressed with his planning. We agreed to meet at his apartment the next week. We would spend some time there and then go to lunch.

He suggested I dress modestly, yet he did say he liked schoolgirl attire. At the time my wardrobe and bank account were pretty limited. I managed to find tights and a mid-length tartan skirt in my closet. I was to look attractive, but not like a sex worker.

Riding the subway there was titillating. I imagined what my

fellow riders would think of me, if they knew where I was going. What I was going to do. I sat with my legs closed, smoothing out my skirt, smiling to myself.

What he wanted sexually was quite specific. He introduced me to his dildo. He told me he wouldn't be able to get an erection, due to his age and health issues, but he could come, if I put that dildo in his ass and sucked his cock at the same time. He was right. It worked. Every time. I would shower afterwards, before we went out to lunch.

Lunch it turned out was more challenging. He was kind to me, but often rude to the waitstaff. I wanted to communicate to them, I'm sorry, I'm one of you. I'm working for tips too. He told me his wife and son hated him. Seeing how he treated the waitstaff at a restaurant, I could imagine what sort of husband and father he was, and why they may truly have hated him.

Yet I saw a different side of him as well. He allowed himself to be vulnerable with me. I saw how much he craved connection, affection and, yes, sex. He told me he was bisexual and had had experiences with men, which was no surprise to me given how he took that dildo. I wondered if he was truly attracted more to men and had never felt safe enough to come out as gay. It felt sad that he possibly still didn't feel safe enough to come out, even in secret. Why have me come over and stick a dildo up his ass, rather than inviting some nice young man who could do the same but with a real cock? And then just send the young man on his way with a check, and skip lunch. No one else would have to know.

I was able to give him at least some of what he craved, without judgment, with genuine affection. He would touch me too and I could easily have an orgasm as I was aroused by the whole scenario. It was naughty and fun and it didn't hurt to walk out with a check for $500.

He only got annoyed at me once, when I left crumbs on the kitchen countertop. This, he said, his wife might notice. He gave me a little scolding. And I found it odd that a few crumbs would be a giveaway. I felt he was taking a huge risk in having me over in the middle of a Wednesday afternoon. What if his wife came home while I was there with his cock in my mouth? That seemed a bigger risk than a dirty kitchen counter.

Once, during our sexy time, he got blood on the quilt. He had some sores on his skin that were bleeding. He was upset by the mess. He immediately wrapped the quilt up and made a call to have someone pick it up and have it specially washed. "It's expensive being rich," he said and laughed at his own joke.

One Wednesday he canceled on me last minute and I called in my cancellation policy. He understood but he got upset. I talked to my therapist about it. "He wants to believe it's not about the money for you," she said. She was right. He admitted it later. He said exactly that. He wanted to feel that I wanted to be there with him. And I had exposed the fantasy. I was learning.

Sex work is about sharing your body for compensation but it is also about creating a fantasy that you are not doing that, that you are sharing because you want to. You enjoy their company. You find them attractive. You are turned on. You truly like them. For me, some of that had to be true. I'm not great at pretending. I've also learned if you look deeply enough at most people, you will find something attractive in them.

I eventually stopped seeing my special friend from the museum. I imagine maybe he came out to himself and found a nice man to visit with and put his dildo aside. Perhaps this allowed him to start liking himself, which meant his wife and son could also stop hating him. And maybe he even began to treat the lunch shift servers with respect. Or none of that is true, but it's the fantasy I've created.

CHAPTER 11
BONDS OF HEALING
My Journey with a Soul in Shadows

Fariba Arabghani

In the dim, sacred space where I work, where the world outside melts away, and what remains is the raw, unfiltered essence of human connection, I stood ready to guide another soul through a transformative journey. This realm, far removed from the chaos and judgment of the outside world, is where I find my purpose, facilitating moments of profound realization and healing. It is in this facilitation that I curate stories that pierce the heart with their weight of sorrow and their potential for liberation.

One such story that remains etched in my heart is the journey I embarked on with Muhammad (a pseudonym to protect his privacy), a Syrian refugee who carried the unbearable weight of survivor's guilt and a malignant sea of unresolved trauma. Muhammad's story is one of profound loss and the indescribable horrors of war. He witnessed the unfathomable—the murder of his family, an event that left deep scars on his psyche. He came to me with a request that was as heart-wrenching as it was healing. Muhammad sought to role-play scenarios where he was blamed for the unthinkable tragedies that had befallen him and his homeland. It was a path he believed would lead him to face and, hopefully, reconcile with the survivor's guilt that shadowed his every step.

Our sessions were built on the sacred foundations of trust and consent, the cornerstones of all the work within the BDSM community. But with Muhammad, there was an added layer of sensitivity and care. Our initial discussions were deep, exploring the boundaries and ensuring that the space we entered together was one of safety, understanding and mutual respect. The role-play was not about reliving trauma but about creating a controlled environment where Muhammad could confront his feelings of guilt and responsibility in a way that was cathartic and, ultimately, healing.

As we delved into the role-play, Muhammad's emotions surfaced with an intensity that was both painful and purifying. Each session was carefully navigated, allowing him to express and experience the depths of his guilt, anger and sorrow within the safe confines of our agreed-on scene. My role as a dominatrix was transformed in these sessions; I was a guide, a witness to his pain, and a bearer of hope that through facing these dark emotions, he could find a path to healing.

In the moments of vulnerability, when the role-play ceased, and the raw, unguarded truth of his pain emerged, I was there to offer support, not as a dominatrix but as a fellow human being capable of compassion and empathy. We ventured together into the depths of his psyche, where the shadows of his past loomed large, and through our sessions, began the delicate work of untangling the guilt from the grief.

Seeing Muhammad confront his deepest fears and begin to untangle the web of guilt and sorrow brought me to tears more than once. His bravery in facing such profound pain reminded me of the transformative power of our work. It moved me deeply, both as a professional and as a human being who has also navigated personal landscapes of pain and recovery. Our sessions became a shared journey, not just his healing but mine as well; they were a reminder of why I do this work, of the deep emotional connections that are possible, and of the mutual transformation that occurs when two people enter a space of such profound trust and vulnerability. Muhammad's journey was one of gradual healing, of learning to live with the memories without being consumed by them. Through our sessions, he began to see that the responsibility for the atrocities he witnessed was not his to bear. The role-play, intense and emotionally charged as it was, provided a mirror for his emotions, allowing him to confront and eventually accept the truth of his innocence in the tragedies that had befallen him.

The path to healing from such profound trauma is neither linear nor predictable. Yet, in the sanctity of our sessions, Muhammad found a space where he could express his deepest sorrows, confront his guilt, and start the long process of healing. Our journey together was a testament to the transformative power of facing one's darkest fears in a space of compassion and understanding.

Reflecting on our sessions, I am continually moved by the trust and openness that clients like Muhammad bring into our shared space. It's a profound privilege to facilitate and witness such incredible personal transformations. Each story of healing, each moment of breakthrough, reinforces my passion and commitment to this work. I feel incredibly fortunate to be able to guide and support individuals on their journeys towards self-discovery and healing. This work is not just a professional path but a profound personal journey that constantly teaches, challenges and enriches my understanding of human resilience and emotional depth.

CHAPTER 12

GARY: MY MILITARY MAN

Tracy Lee

This was my first visit with Gary. We chatted a bit to get acquainted, and through our discussions it came up that he was military, but he was vague about his work. He mentioned having seen horrible things.

I had worked with military men before, but never one as intense as him. In my Full Body Sensual Massage (FBSM) sessions with military men I noticed they would never fully relax. Even though they said they were, the subtle tension in their bodies told another story. Always curious about finding openings for more pleasure, I pondered on what might be going on with these men. On duty, always prepared for danger. But, I'm no threat. How can I get them to stop searching for danger? My first try, I told the client, "There is no danger here. Can you notice that and see if you can relax a bit more?" That worked to a point, but as I fumbled around with a couple other tense clients, I thought again, and the simplest answer came to me.

These men respond to orders, not invitations. So, next time, I eased us into the touch part of the session with some cuddling. I then said, "Look me in the eye," and then forcefully, "Soldier, you are off duty for the next 90 minutes." I had found the recipe that worked.

Gary's eyes got wide, and a sense of wonder and disbelief washed over his face. "Really?" he asked. "Yes," I replied. "Your job now is to just relax, there is nothing for you to do right now." This man, military trained, fearing nothing, got tears in his eyes. I pulled him closer to me and wrapped my arms around him as if he was a child. He wept. Big bawling tears of the child trained out of him to do violence, always to be on-point, follow orders, protect at all costs. To be gifted time off and held lovingly undid this man. What a sweet and precious moment to witness.

Gary practically crawled into my lap. He buried his face in my shoulder, tears wetting my shirt, while I, just a petite pixie, wrapped my arms around this big burly man's shuddering body the best I could. Gary's body was warm against mine, his hair soft and tickly against my face, he smelled of citrus and the out-doors. I held him as if I would never let him go. "Oh, thank you, thank you," he stammered through tears over and over again.

Eventually, his tears abated, and our clinging embrace settled down, but we maintained the nurturing cuddles until the end of the session, never getting him on the massage table at all. This was what he needed most.

I saw Gary two more times after that until work took him away. We were able to get him on the table for that sensual touch session. There weren't any more tears. He said, "Tracy, you don't know how much this means to me." "Tracy, thank you for helping me, loving me. Tracy, you are amazing. Thank you for being you." He shared his appreciation and gratitude of how healing it was for him to take "time-off" with me.

I was so grateful that Gary found the healing he needed and I was part of it. I am continually amazed at the power of touch.

This session with Gary brought that home for me. Even the simplest touch, given with love and compassion, has profound effects. Frequently in my sessions, I struggle with frustration that so many people either have no one in their lives to touch them, or struggle to enjoy it due to an "unwanted touch event." It opens my heart to see tears, hear the stories of these tragedies, and be just a moment in time of healing, witnessing and showing acceptance to my clients. This is why I do this work I love so dearly.

CHAPTER 13

SEX (AS) THERAPY

Court Vox

Before I became a sex and intimacy coach full time, I was a corporate executive with a side hustle, and when I say hustle, I mean it. I was a hustler, an escort, whore, prostitute... Choose your avatar, I revel in all the titles.

My work as an escort led me to what I do now. I recognized that while sex was desired, it was the antidote for larger themes like loneliness, self-hatred, connection, expression, love and creativity. Except, my role was to offer a great experience, not to point out the themes present just beneath the surface.

As I began to transition into coaching, many of my clients became interested in my work and started opening up to me in new and incredibly vulnerable ways.

In one instance, a client I had worked with once previously hired me, alongside three other men, to make him our play toy for the evening. He requested I arrive an hour before them and stay an hour after. His initial request was to be tied up, spanked, flogged and fucked, but as I began offering the experience he had dreamt of, I noticed he wasn't present with me, so I stopped and checked in. He spoke that he wanted to be untied and did not like being spanked or flogged and he just wanted to be bent over and fucked. Easy enough! As I bent him over the very large dark velvet sofa I had a panoramic view of the large space, complete with a roaring fire in the fireplace, floor-to-ceiling glass looking out to the pool and garden. I was in my own cinematic moment and it was sexy.

An hour in, the others arrived and I quickly debriefed them that he was just wanting to be fucked by all of us. We all entered the bedroom and began taking turns on him. The four of us all meaty, muscled and hairy, with beards. Again, a cinematic moment some only dream of having. This man got his wish.

After about an hour, we all came on his chest almost simultaneously (which only happens in porn, most of the time), and lay toppled on one another in a heap of heat, sweat, body hair and breathlessness. And, he was happy.

The other men dressed themselves and said their goodbyes. As I toweled off and put my shorts back on, the man asked if I would sit with him by the fire for a bit. Naturally I accepted, and as he sat next to me, he cuddled up into my arms and lap and I held him. I could feel a tension in him wanting to break free, and so I broke the silence: "How was that for you?"

"It was incredible for me and I'm feeling so much right now," he said.

"If you'd like to share something with me, I will listen," I said.

The man began to share. "When I was in high school I had a boyfriend. We were not out and were both hiding our relationship from our friends and family. It was a different time then and the idea of being gay felt so risky and I felt real fear for my safety and well-being. He, on the other hand, wanted to come out, wanted us to come out together so we could be together, to be free. His desire for this scared me so much that I broke up with him. Not only did I end things with him, I began to ostracize him at school, joining the other kids in teasing him, purposefully and consciously aiming to separate myself from him in all the ways possible, to keep myself from being marked. It felt terrible and powerful all at once. I still loved him, and while I hated myself, I got off on the power I now held over him. It was my twisted way of holding on to us, while protecting myself from harm. He was the faggot and I was the survivor.

One day, I came to school, it was Tuesday, and he wasn't there. Two more days passed and he still did not come to school. In equal parts of relief and grief, his absence began to eat at my stomach. On Friday morning I entered school to a buzz and a flurry of hurried and worried conversations. In a flip off-hand conversation between two girls passing me in the corridor, I heard them say, 'Did you hear Jeffrey died? Yeah, he hung himself.' My heart caved, my eyesight went fuzzy, my legs felt heavy and it was an effort to merely stand, let alone move. I'm not sure how I made it to the bathroom, but I found myself sitting alone in the stall, door shut, and I began to cry silently so no one could hear me. I cried into the sleeve of my sweatshirt to deaden the noise. When I could not cry anymore, I stood up, opened the door, avoided looking at myself in the mirror, exited the bathroom and walked to English class as if nothing had happened. I have been in therapy for the last ten years and was too ashamed to speak about it there. I have been holding this for 20 years and you are the first person I have ever told.

"I have always wanted to experience being fucked by a lot of men, I have always wanted to be free in my sexuality and until now I was not able. I did not think I deserved it, deserved any kind of pleasure or happiness. I've been punishing myself for over 20 years for what I did, and I'm ready to forgive myself."

"I feel very honored that you have shared something so deeply intimate and vulnerable with me. I am so sorry for your loss, and that you have been living with this burden for so long. Is there anything you need from me, anything you'd like me to say?"

"No. I just needed to say it out loud, and I knew you wouldn't judge me."

"I'm not and I won't."

We sat for a bit longer, in the dark, lit only by the large fire in the living room, him cuddled in my chest, quietly crying.

"Let it out. It's alright to cry."

As his whimpers calmed, his tears well laid into my chest hair, he sat up and said, "Thank you for listening. I'm okay. How much do I owe you?"

After settling up and hugging him goodbye, I walked the paces to the large front door, through the garden, past the pool, down the dark, quiet street to my car. I opened the door and sat still, quiet. I slowly began to wail and scream and beat my dash. I cried for him, I cried for myself, I cried for every man who has suffered from having to hide himself. I cried, and yelled until my body felt clean and purged. I started my car and drove myself home.

The man reaches out every once in a while but I have not seen him since then.

While this story is sad, please do not feel sorry for this man as you will only undermine the brave reclamation of himself and his healing through his expression of the erotic and pleasure.

To celebrate him is to celebrate yourself.

CHAPTER 14

NATE'S PENILE CONUNDRUM

Tapping into the Wisdom of the Body

Victoria Angel Heart

I had been seeing my client Nate off and on for seven months when he came to me with a desire to try my integrated modality that merges the Emotional Freedom Technique (tapping) with Conscious Energetic Touch and sexological bodywork practices. If you aren't familiar with those terms, basically he wanted a session where he could find freedom from the emotions that were causing pain in his body, while being held, touched and supported to release the stored trauma.

"Hey Nate! Welcome back." He's just returned from a plant medicine retreat, where he discovered more somatic experiences of trauma he can feel in his body but can't remember happening. He's been questioning if the sexual abuse was real or not for many months, and his intention for this session is to simply be with the physical symptoms in his body.

Before we begin, I invite him to drop into his body and orient himself to the room to feel safe. I know that his sexual trauma presents itself in different ways during every session, so I take extra care to remind him of his agency. "We can go as slow as you need, we can stop at any time, and you are always at choice. I will ask before touching you and you can let me know whenever you change your mind. I will give you suggested phrases while we tap, and you can change them however you need so they feel right to you."

He grins sheepishly, having heard me give this speech at the beginning of every session, and nods in agreement.

"Let's start by making a movie title for what we want to work on today. What would we call this movie?"

"Nate's Penile Conundrum," he says half-jokingly, and we both giggle. "What's the intensity of it from 0 to 10, with 0 being nothing and 10 being the most intense feeling ever?"

"It's about an 8."

"So tell me, what's happening in your body when you think about your penile conundrum?"

"I feel this energy in my genitals that feels both physical and emotional. It doesn't come up during sex, just when I'm meditating or tapping, doing something internal."

"Are you open to describing in more detail where you're feeling sensation and what you're experiencing?"

He tells me that it's an excruciating, torturous pain, and with it comes the shame of being violated and the anger that someone is getting pleasure from his pain.

"It sounds as if you're feeling rage. Does that land?"

"Yes, it's definitely rage!" His brunette curls shake as he agrees with me.

I invite him to start tapping as he talks. Tapping, also known as the Emotional Freedom Technique, is a practice of percussively tapping on the body's acupressure points so that stored-up energy in the body is allowed to move freely through the various meridians. It's like acupuncture without the needles, and has been transformative in my own life and the lives of my clients, so I feel a lot of hope as Nate and I begin to tap.

"Tell me about this rage you're feeling."

He taps on the top of his head, and a stream of thoughts come out.

"I can't act on it, I keep it suppressed or else it'll make things worse, something bad will happen. I don't have the right to express it. I don't feel as if there's anything wrong with me or I have done anything bad. Does this mean something happened to me? Did something really happen to me? Am I just making this up? Do I have a right to think this? I'm afraid because of the uncertainty. Is this really coming from sexual abuse or is it just random pain from somewhere in my body?"

I lead him through tapping on these thoughts, interspersed with the phrases "I am open to loving and accepting myself" and "I deeply and completely love and accept myself." Because Nate has been tapping for a while, these phrases are easy for him to say. I remind him that if at any point they don't feel true, he can say "It is what it is" or "Here and now, I'm okay" instead.

We follow the thoughts and I ask him, "What would happen if that happened? And then what? And then what?" His thoughts become more and more absurd, until it ends with him saying, "And then I would just die! And even if I died of this rage, I can still love and accept myself."

At the end of this round of tapping, I ask him to breathe and check in with the rage.

He looks up, wide-eyed. "It's gone!" We both laugh, always in awe when tapping works so effectively.

"So how about this Penile Conundrum story? What's the intensity now?"

"It's down to about a 3. But something is coming up in reaction to this. I'm feeling some anger. It doesn't want to be belittled."

"It sounds like a part needs to keep its identity. What does it need?"

He begins to tap in between his eyebrows, and takes a deep breath.

As he moves to his temple, he begins to speak, and as he goes through each point, he says, "Reassurance! The amount of pain and suffering is just as significant, regardless of if it happened. It's been four or five years of the most abhorrent torture in my body. I'm afraid that without the story I don't deserve sympathy or compassion anymore—the story gives me more excuses, and it makes me more deserving of love and kindness. Without it I'm a crazy person making up stuff and should just get over it!"

I invite Nate to consider that this part has been protecting him, and doing a great job for several years of making sure that he's receiving support and care to help him feel better. I ask him to reflect on how the part might have been trying to serve him.

I am awed by the insight he shares as he taps and begins to yawn as he speaks. Yawning is a form of off-gassing, where the body releases the pent-up energy that's been stored, so I can tell the tapping is working.

"It's been doing the best it can with the information available. It's been working so hard for me! For a period, whether it's true or not, it gave me hope. It gave me something to work on, a diagnosis that there are treatments for, instead of just having literally nothing or no idea what it could be or where it's from. I respect the tenacity and strength that's there. I love and respect myself."

I feel warm tears stream down my cheeks as I encourage him to give this part the love and kindness it deserves right now.

As his body shakes and yawns, he says, "Do you hear me little part? You're worthy of this love! You're worthy of kindness. I deeply and completely love and accept you."

I check in with him and ask, "What else does this part need to feel safe and supported?"

He looks surprised as he gushes out, "It feels safe and supported right now!"

"Let's add some positive possibilities here. What kind of good code do you want to put in now that we've reduced the intensity of this little part?"

"I'm ready to let this go now. I'm giving myself the support, kindness, love and compassion I've been needing. Turns out I can give it to myself! I love and respect myself. I deeply love and care for you, little part. I'm so proud of what you've been able to do with your creativity and willingness to keep trying new things and your hunger for seeking the truth."

We pause and check in, and he says he's ready to put more positive possibilities in.

"What would you have, do, be or experience if this pain was gone?"

Just asking the question lights up his face! He starts tapping the side of his thumb, and moves down every finger and the side of his hand as he confidently lists what he'd have.

"More energy! I'd be more connected to my family. I'd have time and energy for fun things with my friends, and new hobbies. I'd feel more open, lighter. Going inside my body would be easier. I'd have a lot more sexual enjoyment and feel lighter in my genitals. Even though I have some remaining resistance to this story I could see some benefits of letting this go, so I can love and accept myself, right now."

He exhales deeply and yawns, then looks at me.

"How is the pain in your genitals now?"

"I still feel sensation there but it's not intense or painful. It's dull, unpleasant, like sandpaper on the right-side tip."

"Would you like to shift gears and do some table work? We can explore the sensation you're feeling in your genitals with some self-touch, or I can touch you if you prefer. Our goal will be to bring love, compassion, kindness and support to the place where you feel the dull sensation on the tip. We'll keep tapping the whole time, and I can tap on you if you need your hands. Would you like to try?"

"Yes, I'm open to self-touch for this. But I want to go slow, because it might feel super intense."

I invite him to lie on the table and undress to the level of his comfort, and reassure him that we can go as slow as he needs.

"Can I be in my underwear?"

"Yep! You can have on whatever amount of clothes feels right to you."

I go to wash my hands and let him undress, then knock and re-enter the warm, inviting temple room.

I place my chair about a foot from the table and ask him if he wants me closer, further away or if it is just right.

"That's perfect."

I say, "Place one hand on your heart and one hand on your genitals." He does so, tentatively. "Let's just breathe here together."

After a few moments of breathing, I invite him to start tapping with the hand on his chest and to slowly bring his other hand to the right tip of his penis, where he has been experiencing pain.

His body twitches and he begins to breathe more heavily. I ask him to describe the sensation.

"It's a dull ache now."

We start tapping, and we tap on the possibility that this pain might last forever and it might get so big and be so intense that he might die.

Nate starts to laugh and I can see a change coming over his body.

"Is it okay if I put my hand over your hands and my other hand can tap for you?" I ask. He agrees.

We do a round of tapping on accepting this pain without the story and just letting it be what it is, while also loving and accepting it.

He takes a deep breath inside at the end of that round, then he asks tentatively, "Can I take my underwear off?"

"Yes, whatever feels comfortable. You can also put it back on whenever you like."

In seven months of working together, I have never seen him naked. We have done so much work together, but this is the first time he has felt ready to be on the table without clothes. I feel myself beaming with pride that he feels safe enough to take this big step with me.

I give him space to remove his clothes, then I keep tapping on his chest after he lies back on the table, nude.

His hands slowly make their way to his genitals, and his

thumbs begin to softly stroke his cock. As it gets hard, he begins to breathe with an intense energy that makes his body shake.

"Can I keep tapping on you?"

"Yes," he says, "I'd love that."

As we breathe and tap, I invite him to open to the possibility of being with the pain without any story, just as sensation. We go through a few rounds of tapping and his body noticeably begins to soften, his jaw unclenches, and his breathing relaxes.

"What if you give yourself the support, kindness, love and compassion you were needing when you were a child? What if you infuse it into your penis with every breath through the energy coming out of your fingers?"

We tap, and he begins to melt. His erection fades and his whole body softens. I ask him if he is ready to infuse some positive possibilities in where the old stories used to be. When he is ready, he taps and creates these affirmations, which brings me to tears.

"I give myself the possibility of intense pleasure. I am pain free. My body deserves my love. I am available for deeper levels of pleasure now. It's safe to let go of the story and the anger. It's safe to be calm, to rest and relax."

I ask him to give himself a hug and let these affirmations sink in as our time together comes to a close. He puts his clothes back on and returns to his chair, glowing and grinning from ear to ear.

"How is the penile conundrum now?"

"It's nearly gone, I'd say it's significantly reduced, down to a 1. It's almost not there anymore. Wow!"

With that, our session comes to a close, and he walks out

with less pain in his body and more emotional freedom than he's had in five years of trying various healing modalities.

This story explains why I love integrating tapping into hands-on work with clients. Even though I don't even touch his genitals, his ability to be naked, touch himself and feel safe enough to keep tapping through the process allows more to be released in his body than either modality could do on its own.

CHAPTER 15

THE HEALING POWER OF KINK

Emme Witt-Eden

C hristopher called early on Saturday, asking to see me at noon. He was clean and respectful and he always tipped. In short, he was a great client. For this reason, I accepted his last-minute session request. We had a good rapport, and I was happy to share my energy with him. It also didn't surprise me that he called on a Saturday. He once told me that Sundays were for church, Wednesdays were for Bible study, but Saturdays were for pain.

Christopher was what is known in popular "dominatrix vernacular" as a *pain slut*, or someone who enjoys being tortured. He didn't like to be humiliated; he wasn't into that. Because I only played safely and sanely, within the parameters of consent, sticking with Christopher's turn-ons was never a problem. I didn't want to humiliate him, calling him names or engaging him in other degrading activities, if that wasn't something he derived pleasure from in some way.

He arrived at the dungeon at noon sharp on a motorcycle, clad in leather. Once inside, he shed the jacket and pants and knelt before me, naked. I cuffed him to the St. Andrew's Cross, arms overhead, legs spread wide. In that position, he gave me carte blanche to do pretty much whatever I wanted to him. Well, anything but humiliation.

Picking up a cat-o'-nine-tails, I pelted his butt with it, listening as the leather strips hit his skin. Then, after his behind was a rosy pink, welts blooming on his epidermis, I turned him around and got to work on his penis and testicles. Using clamps, weights and a violet wand, I meted out the cock and ball torture. As I did, his penis hardened and quivered. Clearly, he was getting off on this.

I continued to work him over, keeping to activities that I knew he liked (impact play and genital torture). This was why I believe he saw me repeatedly. I curated a specific session based on activities I believed he enjoyed. And yes, though I might torture him, I never pushed him beyond his limits.

He once shared that another pro-domme did disrespect his consent by tying him down and caning him till he bled. She wouldn't stop even when he begged her to. She also engaged him in quite a bit of verbal humiliation. He said the experience was traumatizing—re-traumatizing.

Christopher was open about having grown up in a strict, fundamentalist Christian household where, sadly, there was physical and emotional abuse. This was why he frequented dominatrixes, he said. I know this is a stereotype, that submissives have been abused in their childhoods and therefore seek out the same treatment as adults, but this *was* Christopher's case. However, this other pro-domme abused his consent and put him in that traumatized space again. In contrast, with me, he felt as if he could transcend that trauma.

Being tortured by me was healing because Christopher felt that he regained power over his past in our sessions. In being the one to request said punishment—and having his limits respected by me when he did—he felt strong again. And, of course, experiencing this torture mixed with erotic release was also freeing.

Because of my experience with clients like Christopher, I've been happy about the numerous mainstream essays and scientific papers that have been published in the recent past exploring the therapeutic benefits of kink. Participants in BDSM and fetish play are capable of healing from trauma by willingly enduring physical and emotional discomfort. Through structured role-play scenarios, they revisit painful memories in a space where they feel secure and supported. In such a context, some submissives are actually able to rewire their nervous systems, "rewriting" their traumatic histories in a scenario where they feel that they finally have agency. Engaging in BDSM activities, such as being bound by ropes, subjected to whipping or other forms of consensual torture, can also lead individuals to discover empowerment by embracing their vulnerabilities.

Thankfully, the medical community has also revised its stance on kink. Having a fetish or deriving sexual satisfaction from consensual masochism or sadism is no longer considered a mental illness by many mainstream psychologists. In the latest edition of the *Diagnostic and Statistical Manual of Mental Disorders (DSM-5)*, the standard classification of mental disorders used by mental health professionals in the United States, the American Psychiatric Association asserted that most individuals who engage in kinky activities—such as cross-dressing, fetishism and BDSM—do not have a mental disorder.

As a professional BDSM practitioner, I have welcomed such a shift in the societal perceptions of kinky people. If submissives are no longer deemed mentally unfit, then dominatrixes are also no longer stereotyped as heartless man-haters with unresolved emotional problems. Instead, today's pro-domme is increasingly viewed as a compassionate provider who can contribute positively to her submissives' personal growth. Finally, society is waking up to the fact that, in much part during our sessions, dominatrixes assume a caregiving role.

In my experience, I've often felt like a sort of shaman whose job is to take my clients on journeys to the most forbidden realms of their psyche. During a curated experience, I lead my submissives to experience taboo parts of themselves and even make peace with them. However, in saying this, there are limits to how much I can heal every client who darkens the doorway of my dungeon. Sometimes, I have to prioritize my mental health over my clients' experiences. Not all clients are willing to be helped or healed.

I took pity on José. He was younger than most of my clients, only 23 years old. As he was in college, and I was the first dominatrix he had ever had a session with, I allowed him to see me at a deeply discounted rate. He seemed very submissive during our initial phone interview. His kinks were for ball-busting (being hit or kicked in the testicles) and heavy trampling (being walked and even jumped on while lying flat). I hoped I could give José a great experience, and, apparently, I did, as he came back to see me again and again. But unfortunately, he would ultimately turn on me.

After numerous sessions, he suddenly stopped calling. He didn't contact me again until a few months later, giving me a cryptic story about having spent time in some kind of Christian "rehab." He begged for a heavy whipping session, which

I facilitated, but at the end of the meeting, he changed his tune, suddenly declaring that he hadn't liked what we'd done in session. He demanded a refund.

Though I felt very annoyed about this, especially because I had already given him a deeply discounted "student rate," I returned his money and thought that was the end of him. It wasn't. A week later, José called again, apologizing profusely, saying he would pay me double if I would take him back. I'm a dominant, and we hadn't ended on a good note. He hadn't ask for his refund respectfully and the session concluded in a heated argument. But, I took pity on him and let him come back to see me.

We had a few more sessions, but then he did the same thing. He asked for another refund, shouting at me as he did. When I said that this time I wouldn't refund his money as I now saw this was a game, he threatened to out me to my neighbors and have my business shut down. Maybe he would even call the police on me.

José is one of those clients whom I couldn't help and who was even intent on hurting me. Why? I believe that he was filled with shame about his kinks, which was only exacerbated by whatever Christian "recovery" program he'd been in. He wasn't like Christopher, who engaged in BDSM play to heal from his strict religious background. I think José's faith just contributed to his self-hatred, and he took this hatred out on me.

Meetings with clients need to be based on mutual respect. Once I figured out the extent of José's shame and how he was now going to use this dynamic to get free sessions from me and, worse, threaten me while doing so, I had to protect myself by not seeing him anymore. I should never have agreed to another session with José after the first time he insulted me and asked for a refund, but I did because I thought I could help him. During our initial sessions, he always voiced how much calmer he felt afterwards. But now, not only did I believe I couldn't help him anymore, but I felt as if I was putting my entire existence into jeopardy by continuing to meet with him.

It wasn't just that José could ruin my business by getting me evicted from my studio, he could entangle me in legal difficulty. I could get arrested and end up with an offense on my record. By this point, I felt as if my mental health was also being harmed by José. Even being in his presence felt like sharing his bad energy, and that was taking its toll on me. This isn't to say that I also didn't fear that he might ultimately hurt me physically. In my opinion, José didn't need a "dominatrix therapist," he needed an actual therapist.

In the end, I had to prioritize my own mental health and physical safety over his "well-being." I wish I could say that José was my only client like this. I can't. I've had other clients play similar games with me, showing they had zero respect for me either as a professional or a person.

I've been insulted by clients when I've upset them in some way, typically because I wouldn't agree to participate in a certain activity with them in session. Consent is the cornerstone of any healthy BDSM scene and it's not just the submissive who gets to have limits, the dominant does, too. Although I've never been attacked by a client in session, I've had to terminate meetings with clients who didn't follow the rules, especially those who demanded I disregard my own boundaries to fulfill their sexual needs. Luckily, as a professional dominant, I'm in a better position to manage such clients, as part of my role is to re-establish my dominance in any dynamic with a client. This position of dominance inherently grants me a degree of protection compared to other types of providers, given that my clients typically adopt submissive roles. Nevertheless, I've still encountered disrespect from clients and have felt compelled to take extra precautions to ensure my safety.

In sharing the stories of the negative experiences I've had with a few bad clients, I don't want to perpetuate yet another damaging stereotype that sex workers are constantly being victimized. We're not. I also don't want to make it seem as if I haven't been able to help many other clients throughout the years. Some of my clients have told me that, because of our sessions, they've had better relationships with women. And for those who are suffering in their marriages, maybe because their wives refuse to have sex with them, I have also provided an intimate space for them to feel close to a woman.

I did this for a client named Barry, who wanted to worship a woman as her "kissing slave." For this session, he requested that I lay face down on a surface while he lightly kissed my entire body. I know this doesn't sound very "dominant" of me, but I thought the session seemed harmless enough—and it was. Not only that, I helped Barry. Through our session, I believe he experienced an intimate situation with a woman without feeling that he was cheating on his wife, who had health issues and was no longer able to have sex with him.

I've also helped clients with loneliness. I did this for a man named Jason, who shared his battle with depression after one of our sessions. When he asked if I could hug him at the close of our meeting, I obliged, enveloping Jason's form in my arms. As he rested his head on my shoulder, I could sense the fragile tremors coursing through his body. About three minutes later, he raised his head and whispered, "You have no idea how much I needed that." When he finally left the dungeon that day, he left less burdened by his angst and insecurities. I believe our session was therapeutic for him, as my sessions have been with other clients.

I gave emotional support to a man when his wife caught him dressing up in women's clothing. When she told him she wanted a divorce, I became a listening board as he was going through this tragic life experience. Sometimes, for my clients, just having me there to tell them that I don't think their fantasy is sick, that they aren't crazy for having the fetishes they do, that there isn't anything wrong with them, is enough.

CHAPTER 16

ARCHETYPES AND THE ENERGETIC POLARITY

Sex Work is Healing Work

Sadie Hudson

A flower in bloom carries the seeds of its successor; only in death is this potential released.

—SADIE HUDSON

Author's note on names and certain details: These have been changed or omitted to protect the confidentiality and anonymity of my clients and/or myself.

Author's note on language: This piece is an exploration of the polarity between masculine and feminine sexual-spiritual energies. The stories herein refer to specific men and women, as well to "men and women" in the socio-cultural-historical sense, so those terms and associated pronouns are used where appropriate. However, these energies are not gender-specific, and gender-neutral pronouns have been incorporated where possible.

BECOMING: THE HIGH PRIESTESS OF PLEASURE

It was May 2022 and I was nearing my three-year anniversary as an online sex worker, where I'd specialized in one-on-one services such as sexting, private cam shows and online girl-friend experience. That spring, I decided to take the plunge and become an escort, also known as a full-service sex worker.

To set the stage a little, I was emerging from a two-year stint of involuntary isolation, initially due to Covid restrictions, and later to protect an immune-compromised family member with a terminal illness. I'd developed a spiritual practice to cope with the extreme social deprivation, with a focus on Divine Feminine energies. When I re-entered the world that May, my practice was two to three hours per day. As a result, I was primed to embody the feminine principle in my work, something that would not have been possible without the aforementioned spiritual devotion. One of the other gifts of my spiritual foundation as an escort has come in the form of transpersonal insights into our sexual natures.

Some of these insights were the product of patterns I observed in my clients, archetypes I've named The Sensualist, The Lover and The Lion. These archetypes represent my clients' sexual DNA, if you will—a blueprint of their sexual nature which tells us something about their needs, how they interact sexually with others, what drives them, and what pains them.

As the yin to my clients' yang, these experiences also called forth archetypical aspects in me. My Covid cloistering prepared me to embody these energy forms, but without sexual sovereignty, I could not have done so professionally (that is, repeatedly and consistently). Not only would I have not had the necessary growth, but my prior conditioning would have stood in my way.

In my journey to sexual sovereignty, two challenges have been surprisingly difficult to overcome: putting myself at the center of my own sexual experiences, and learning to claim and enact my power. It turns out there's a glass ceiling in the bedroom, too, one I had internalized. At first, I was entirely unconscious of how much my conditioning had placed my role and experience as secondary to the man in the room. By default, his desires, his fantasies and his pleasure gave impetus to what unfolded; when I looked for evidence of sexual volition of my own, I found nothing. Even the encounters themselves were defined by the linear trajectory favored by men, one that begins with an erection and ends with ejaculation. It was utterly foreign to me to be the powerful protagonist, the one who defines the terms of engagement.

Connecting to my sexuality brought me into wholeness, and I was dedicated to serving the truth it contained. On the other side of the glass ceiling, I found a deep sense of belonging to myself. Little did I know, this subtle inner shift would have outsized effects on my outer world. What delighted me then, and what delights me now, is that by putting myself at the center of my own sexual experiences, I unlocked in men an aspect I craved but only intuitively knew existed.

VENUS AND THE SENSUALIST

As a newly minted escort, I took to the work naturally and easily. The majority of my bookings were downright amazing—magical, electric, meaningful, fun. Many were transformative, some even transcendent. More often than not, they had arche-typical undertones.

One of the most exalted experiences I had in this vein was with Patrick. In his mid-sixties with kind eyes, a burly stature, deep voice and a quick laugh, Patrick was a manly man who made good company. His unruly chestnut curls were surprisingly soft. During the 90-minute booking, he drank in the experience, savoring it like a rare vintage of wine.

Nothing was rushed and everything was intentional. Patrick is the epitome of a client archetype I call The Sensualist. These clients adore the Venus archetype in women—soft skin, voluptuous bodies, enticing curves and intoxicating tastes and scents. They are particularly attuned to the sensory aspects of a sexual encounter and appreciate sensory accompaniments, such as mood lighting and chocolate. They are generous lovers and want to savor every moment with a slow, deliberate pace. Sensualists enjoy the experience of a woman.

As I stood before Patrick and peeled off my dress, a gasp escaped his lips.

"Oh my God," he whispered, his starry eyes widening in an expression I call "boob face"—a mix of awe, delight and anticipation.

I sat down beside him and laid back on the bed, inviting him to join me. He placed one hand on my shin and leaned onto his other elbow to recline next to me. He began caressing my leg as his eyes feasted on my nude body.

"Your skin is so soft!" he gushed, expressing self-consciousness at his rough hands, about which I reassured him. Patrick gave me no roughness; what I felt in his touch, in fact, was reverence. He caressed me with intention, appreciation and adoration; with love, even. When his exploring hand reached my hip, he paused to look up at me.

"Can I touch your belly?" He sounded apprehensive and I sensed that he'd previously been rebuked for his adoration of plump women's midsections.

"Absolutely!" I said emphatically, looking up at him and smiling wide. I reached over to begin caressing his back as his hand moved to my soft, round stomach. Again, he gasped. In his voice was pure rapture: "You have a woman's body," he softly declared, emitting non-verbal utterances of amazement.

Patrick and I did not have intercourse; I don't even think we kissed. He declined all attempts for me to reciprocate the pleasure or shift the focus onto him, saying that, medically, he probably couldn't handle too much excitement. As he was leaving, he confessed to me that his recent life-saving surgery had failed and he would be facing death in the not-too-distant future. He'd given himself the experience of "enjoying a woman's body" so that he could cherish it as his health declined.

Although a gift to himself, our time together gifted me with the experience of witnessing and receiving a pure and potent form of The Sensualist manifestation of the masculine principle. Without my prior devotion to awakening the Divine Feminine in me, I could not have been the provider Patrick needed.

In my life prior to this, I'd leaned heavily into my naturally abundant masculine energies: partly because it's an advantage in our society, partly for protection, and partly to sidestep the problem of my highly sexual nature. Over time, this led me to neglect and abuse my body, devalue daily pleasures, and work myself to the point of breaking. I lost my connection to life. I had abandoned the feminine principle in me, and in so doing, had disconnected from the feminine element in life itself. What's more, my natural overabundance of masculine energy led me to favor sexual encounters that were primal, intense and highly combustible. Decades of living with this energetic asymmetry had rendered me unable to do the things Patrick needed me to do—to relish in being adored, to sink deeply into a moment, to find delicious intensity in a pace that would have previously left me feeling frustrated and bored.

Many of my Sensualist clients have difficulty finding partners who are able to embody the feminine principle of receptivity. The de-feminization I underwent in my own life has played out in Western societies over a couple of thousand years, and most people suffer from it to some degree or another. It's difficult not to, because to do otherwise is to swim against the current. This made Patrick's need for feminine softness a rarity. Every time I am called to embody Venus energies with a client, the feminine principle in me is healed. This characterization surprises people, and it surprises them further that the healing is mutual.

FREYA AND THE LOVER

Four years earlier, in 2018, my new sexual power was lighting up my life. I was learning how to be the agent of my own desire, which was my first challenge on the road to sexual sovereignty. Even in the early days of my second awakening, I felt inspired by the idea of sexual sovereignty for women. I saw how it was bringing me into the deepest alignment and highest form of integrity I had ever known. I believed that if my personal transformation were to occur on a cultural, or even international, level, where a critical mass of sexually sovereign women were reached, it would heal much of what is broken within and between us, just as it had for me. Perhaps what most galvanized this belief for me was not my own liberation and re-alignment, but witnessing its impact on my relationships with men.

In 2018, men transformed overnight. Initially, I noticed things like getting immediate responses to my messages, or being pursued for months and months (which became years), sometimes by people I'd slept with, other times by people I'd only texted, with efforts that continued well after I stopped responding. At the age of 39, my era of irresistibility—which is still ongoing—had begun. Over time, however, my observations became less personal and more archetypical. I noticed that by claiming my sexual power and embodying the feminine principle in a new way, I created a space where men could engage with me in a new way. This brought me my first experiences with an archetype of the masculine principle that I call The Lover. I've had the great fortune of experiencing The Lover many times, and I don't mind saying I have a favorite, who you will meet shortly.

What's unique about Lovers is that their fundamental sexual orientation is to serve the pleasure of their partner. To be clear, there is nothing subservient or submissive about Lovers; they wholly reside in the masculine principle. Rather, these are men whose greatest pleasure comes from seeing the untamed feminine principle unleashed, and they facilitate this by selflessly serving her desire. They love seeing a woman in the throes of genuine pleasure, to see her act on her desires and embody the full power of her sexuality. They are captivated by it, in awe of it. Lovers are invigorated by the wild, chaotic nature of the feminine principle and will find satisfaction in providing the container for this exquisite manifestation.

Much like The Sensualist, Lovers adore women simply for being women. The difference between them is that while The Sensualist's greatest pleasure is the experience of a woman, The Lover's pleasure is derived from that of their partner.

Michael, A.K.A. my favorite, knew how to bring intensity without pain, a hallmark of The Lover that has unfortunately been devalued in an era marked by Fifty Shades and eroticized violence. He had a masterful understanding of my body and my pleasure; he not only knew where and how to touch me, but could read my body's responses and adjust accordingly. An erotic entanglement between two Lovers is like dancing among the stars; the two energies chase and play with each other, spiraling toward union as Self gradually dissolves. As the embodiment of the feminine principle in that encounter, I poured all of my energy into him. With the generosity of his attentiveness, he was more than capable of containing it.

Michael and I generated so much heat that the mirrors in the room were foggy; our bodies dripped with sweat. As we merged, the emotional tone shifted with our energies, producing moments of belly laughter, cry-gasms and animalistic fucking. After an encounter like that, you feel as if you've traveled to another dimension, and this was no exception. Michael and I returned to Earth after the beautiful experience of a shared orgasm (my third and his first), leaving us both glowing, cleansed and invigorated.

What The Lover understands is something that science has barely touched on: women's bodies contain a galaxy of pleasure. By serving this capacity, The Lover unlocks new dimensions of pleasure that he can only access with a willing partner. This reality is echoed in sweat ceremony teachings I received from a nêhiyawak (Cree) Elder, where the women were instructed not to participate if we were menstruating. The Elder explained that it would be like "mixing powers," akin to throwing an electric appliance into the bathtub.

"Women don't need these ceremonies to connect to the Creator," he said. "It is men who need these ceremonies."

Just as we don't need ceremonies (or men) to connect to Spirit through our innate sexual energies, we also don't need men to unlock our Divine betrothal of limitless pleasure. Lovers seem to understand this, at least subconsciously. Rather than feeling threatened by it, The Lover is inspired to serve it. And perhaps that is what is so perverse about what mainstream porn has become—not the surgical lighting, fakery or defaulting to roughness, but the entire premise of women serving men's pleasure. If you google "what's the word for getting pleasure from giving pleasure?" you will see evidence of Lovers in our midst, searching for the word that defines them.

Even without a word for it, encountering a woman who has learned to be sexually self-focused will spark recognition in The Lover. This is what made men relentlessly chase me during the chrysalis stage of my sexual sovereignty journey. All of those men were Lovers, and their hunger for my energy was insatiable. Contrary to what our culture tells us about desirability, it seems that a sexually potent and powerful middle-aged woman has the gravitational force of a planet and shines just as brightly.

Although not as alienated as Lions (who we'll discuss next) or forlorn as Sensualists, Lovers still have no name for their nature, see no reflection of themselves in mainstream porn clips, and are misunderstood as cuckolds or submissives. But what's beautiful about Lovers is what's beautiful about a man with purpose—that they may be so inspired to serve that they will fuck themselves to the point of exhaustion to satisfy their slutty, cock-hungry, demon-goddess of a partner.

LILITH AND THE LION

The "second awakening" is my personal term for the midlife sexual peak; it's the second time in the life span that sexual energy rises to the fore. Just like our first awakening at puberty, it's an experience that arouses new knowledge in us. Or at least, that's what it did for me. The knowledge I gained brought me to the precipice of not only an entirely new path, but a new way of being.

This transformation had mobilized me with the imperative to reconcile all that I had known with what I now knew. Deep into my second awakening, I was asking myself panoramic questions. How many times, and in how many ways, have I been trained to abandon my sexuality? I thought back to grade 4 when, at the age of nine, I got my first period and started wearing a bra. That's when people started calling me a slut. The first time it happened, it was a group of girls who had ganged up on me at recess, chanting "Sadie is a slut! Sadie is a slut!" and clapping their hands with each syllable.

Then there was the boy from grade 6 who approached me with a list in hand, brandishing his evidence. "This is a list of all the boys that like you. That means you're a slut," he declared, pushing the list at me while refusing to let me see it. "Why do you want to see it?" he demanded. "See! You're a slut!"

Nothing prepares you for being seen and treated as a sex object before reaching double digits in age. But, being seen and treated as a sex object from childhood does prepare you to go full warrior mode when the second awakening comes. But before I could heed the call to adventure, I had to slay the dragon: over three decades of being socialized to the Eve ideal.

My second awakening pivoted on a desire to get right with my sexuality, once and for all. I'd always been highly sexual, and as a GenX female, that was problematic. Given my social conditioning and Judeo-Christian cultural inheritance, I could not have been more shocked to find that trust-falling into my sexuality led me straight to God(dess). Through Her I learned that pleasure is my birthright, and my sexuality is a legitimate, distinct and significant dimension of being.

Claiming my sexuality and harnessing the life-force energy it begets has made me powerful: wild and untameable. I now know who and what I am—a sacred, human being who was given the gift of being highly sexual. Part of what motivates my work is my desire to share this freedom and self-acceptance with others.

In my five years as a sex worker, I've encountered many colleagues who identify as being highly sexual. We joke about the "slut to whore" pipeline, which is really a story about being confronted with, and then confronting, oppressive social mores about female sexuality. I empathize with the many "civilian" women (an industry term for non-sex workers) I encounter who are bound by this oppression; I know first-hand how deeply embedded it is, and how threatening it is to confront. While that confrontation is well under way culturally, there is a parallel—and I believe related—process that is binding men, or rather, leading men to bind themselves.

Although arising from a mix of individual and cultural factors, a common impetus for this self-oppression centers on the #MeToo movement, which exposed how normalized and pervasive it was to sexually harass and assault women. During #MeToo, men everywhere were confronted with evidence that the greatest threat in many women's lives is men. This has disproportionately affected highly sexual men who are also what I'll call post-feminist men; they want equality in their relations with women, from household chores to orgasm parity. Such men have been unable to reconcile their sexual natures with their desire to be safe, respectful partners to women. They worry that it's their sexuality itself—their alignment with the masculine principle—that is the problem. For my highly sexual clients, it seems the younger the man, the more likely, and the more deeply, he's been affected.

My client Shan was so deeply affected by this inner conflict that he was unable to make love to his former partner. Not only did he struggle emotionally and psychologically with being sexual, but at just 26 years old, he also suffered from erectile dysfunction.

Shan came from a culture where men's entitlement to sex was seen as a given, and where manhood was demonstrated in part through sexual conquest. Shan recognized these attitudes in the #MeToo stories he'd heard and wanted no part of such behavior; he'd also empathized with the women of his youth, whom he witnessed suffering as a result of these norms. The problem for Shan was that he was highly sexual; he had tried to "opt out" of sexuality, but it just wasn't working.

Shan embodied the client archetype I call The Lion, whose highly sexual nature is expressed in passionate acts of sexual intimacy, but is also channeled into things such as achievement, leadership, excellence and service. As lovers, the highly sexual nature of a post-feminist Lion is embedded within their social context; they want to do sex with someone, not to someone. They are drawn to similarly powerful partners, moved by a combination of primal sexual energy and interpersonal intrigue.

In the primal dimension, Lions have what I call "beast mode," which is a state of unrestrained desire that is thrilling and delicious to receive. The Lover also has a "beast mode," but rather than arising as a primal response to curves and cleavage, for The Lover it is activated in response to his partner's vocalizations of pleasure; it is an act of service. When The Lion goes into beast mode, they seek to overtake their lover; they find completion and fulfillment in being received and responded to by the Lioness, who yearns to be overtaken so that they may fulfill their deepest desire: to surrender. What Lions need—and what Shan needed—is a sexually sovereign partner who can be trusted to give voice to their boundaries, desires and hard limits without delay.

What had paralyzed Shan, in addition to the internalized shame and guilt he felt on behalf of all men, was trying to play both sides of the equation in a sexual encounter, resulting in him being over-responsible for his partner's boundaries, safety and pleasure. This was compounded by the fact that he had not experienced a sexually sovereign partner and therefore could not fully count on his partner's commitment to upholding their own boundaries. For Lions to feel safe, they need to know that Lionesses will not hesitate to roar when they have something to say. Without that assurance, The Lion's desire to overtake becomes an ethical and moral quandary.

The idea of men feeling sexually unsafe is borderline taboo in contemporary society, yet I have seen an epidemic of this among both GenZ men and highly sexual, but socially conscientious, men of all ages. One of the underlying problems is that these men are largely encountering women who have been socialized to the Eve ideal. Eve, widely believed to be Adam's first wife, was actually the successor to Lilith, the first woman who was fashioned from the soil, just like Adam. Adam and Lilith had a disagreement about who would be on top during sex, a metaphor for whose sexual power would be honored and whose would not. Lilith chose her sexuality over her mate, something women have been actively discouraged from doing ever since.

To uphold the Eve ideal, we cannot be directly sexual because doing so revokes our "good girl" status and we face the risk of banishment, like Lilith (and if you think "banishment" is hyperbole, consider how society treats and talks about sex workers). Eve is expected to be at least a little unwilling at all times. Even with her husband, sex is a duty, not a shared pleasure. Such socialization instills in us a deeply embedded belief that our sexuality is for men, and even if we don't consciously uphold these ideas, it still shows up as things such as the orgasm gap or the belief that sex begins with an erection and ends with ejaculation. This severs us from our sexual power and rules out any notion of sexual agency. Without these things, The Lioness has no roar.

But what The Lion needs is Lilith The Lioness—someone who will forsake everything, even Eden, for their sexual integrity, who will refuse to be subservient and is capable of demonic rage when wronged. With Lilith, you always know where you stand. With Eve, you never really know for sure. I would argue that even Eve doesn't know where she stands because she was designed to be incomplete on her own; her completion is to be found in her roles as a wife and mother. Not only that, but she is literally a derivative of Adam, being fashioned from his rib. The aspects of Lilith that were left out in the making of Eve are the very aspects that The Lion both seeks and needs.

Historically, Lion men have not struggled because sexual sovereignty for men has been a given. The problematic aspects of this aside, it's meant that they have been the rightful claimants of their sexuality; there is no future partner for whom they ought to save it. It's meant that "male sexuality" is held as a valid construct; there are no scientists debating whether or not it exists. It's been understood that there is an imperative behind this aspect of their nature, and men have been given license to honor that imperative. There is no corollary for women—no time in a girl's life where she learns to wield her sexual power or become acquainted with her sexual energy, no understanding that she will come into her power and her pleasure as a rite of passage, no allowances made for her exploration, no validation of her needs. The notion of "female sexuality" barely exists, if at all, which makes the journey to sexual sovereignty one without a map or established territory.

Although Lioness women have been alienated from their true natures for thousands of years, Lion men are now facing similar self-alienation due to shifts in culture and consciousness.

But for both Lions and Lionesses, the way home is through inner alignment. I have encountered many men who think (or hope) they can sexually liberate their Eve partners—they can't. Liberation is an inside job, and it starts with cutting the ties that bind us. Only then can we align with our true nature.

However, the gift of this misalignment is that it is painful and disturbing. We may find ourselves depleted from being out of integrity, or that the misalignment spills over into other areas of life, with nothing quite working right. We may have difficulty sleeping, or tend toward extremes with hobbies or other pleasures in an attempt to divert our sexual energy into other things. We may also try, like Shan and I both did, to switch it off altogether. And we will try anything and everything, because the alternative is terrifying. But for highly sexual people such as Shan and me, the only answer is sexuality from a place of wholeness.

THE HEALING JOURNEY

Many of us struggle with sex and sexuality for myriad reasons, but understanding the ties that bind us allows us to have compassion for ourselves and for each other. We have all been bound by a culture that profoundly misunderstands sexuality, with little to no guidance on how to set ourselves straight. But for me and many of my clients, the healing process begins with identifying the sources of suffering—the impositions that we internalize as truth.

This process not only frees us to align with our true nature, but restores our own powers of discernment. Rather than taking on ready-made truths, we have direct experience that shows us what Truth looks like, feels like and sounds like. I know I am making spectacular claims here—that sexuality, or sexual energy, can connect us to Truth—but I believe it not only has this capacity, but that's also part of its purpose.

Sexuality is often cast as an optional aspect of our natures, or at the very least, something we ought to be able to transcend if we are mature enough. In reality, sexuality is a body-mind-heart-spirit phenomenon, offering a chance to deeply connect with ourselves, with others and with our power as creators. One of the gifts of sexual energy, in addition to Truth, is that it is life-force energy, or creation energy; as such, we may use it to heal, transform, create or transcend. That is why our most important sexual relationship is not with our partners, but with ourselves.

I have found that the more sexual energy a person has, the more critical the autoerotic relationship becomes because, without it, there is no alignment. Alignment comes from learning to recognize, and then incorporate, feedback from body, mind, heart and/or spirit as we engage with sexuality. Alignment serves a two-fold purpose. One, it keeps us in integrity. Sexual energy is powerful, and with power comes responsibility. Integrity is how I measure my adherence to the maxim to do no harm to self or other, which guides both my professional and personal sexual endeavors. Without integrity, it's difficult to direct an abundance of sexual energy toward our highest good.

The second function of alignment is wayfinding. By finding alignment in the autoerotic relationship, we can then use direct experience with sexual life-force energy to finally come home to our true nature. Being in alignment is what allows us to trust what we are experiencing and recognize higher truth when it comes. The outcomes of this process are personal and individual. For me, it was trust-falling into my sexuality to find Goddess, being inspired to serve the sexual sovereignty of women, and feeling called to serve as a sex worker by sharing my inner freedom and self-acceptance with others. The key to unlocking your true nature is in the alignment of your body-mind-heart-spirit sexuality, your energetic home.

But homecoming isn't the end, it's the beginning. Here I have presented two options—the exploration of archetypes and playing with the masculine-feminine polarity—as ways the sovereign sexual being may explore. When the masculine-feminine sexual and spiritual polarity is activated, it brings both participants into wholeness and alignment, which is profoundly healing and transformative. Each time this happens for me, it feels as if the world is set right in some small way.

Working with archetypes offers us a way to understand something essential about ourselves, but with a narrative that connects us to the intersubjective and transpersonal dimensions of the human experience. I use archetypes to connect more deeply to my partners and clients, while linking my story to that of countless others across time and space. On the journey of sexual sovereignty, the familiar forms of archetypes help to both describe and navigate an undefined landscape.

Regardless of the path you choose or where it takes you, you can count on pleasure, desire and intuition to light your way.

CHAPTER 17

BUSH FOR SALE

BD White

I did a brief stint as a cam girl and a dirty underwear sales-woman, but did I ever tell you about the time I sold my bush for $60? It was pretty cut and dry—the man wanted my pubes, some pictures and a video of the shaving process. I used electric clippers, it was quite spicy. I felt a little bad about the actual volume of pubes, but figured some was better than none. A week later he let me know via email that he had received the package and that it felt so good to hold my bush in his hands. It smelled so good. It felt so soft.

He shared that he missed pubes because his beloved wife was undergoing cancer treatments and had lost all of her hair to the chemo. I was used to clients who were married but chose to never pry. When it came to sex work, I sometimes questioned the ethics of my participation in activities that may have been outside the confines of someone else's marriage. I ultimately concluded that it was not my business (trusting that my clients had either worked out issues of consent with their partners or were prepared for the fallout when their browsing histories came to light). What stuck with me about this one, though, was the way he spoke about his wife in relation to our agreement. He was devoted to her.

He didn't seem to feel guilt over our transaction but made it very clear that his rationale for the purchase was so that he could tend to the parts of him that needed bush to feel satiated, without causing his wife any additional pain by letting her know how much he missed her body hair. We never spoke again. The man just needed some pubes.

CHAPTER 18

LOOKING FOR A LITTLE ROMANCE

Maya

The lady in red is dancing with me, cheek to cheek. There's nobody here, it's just you and me, it's where I want to be, but I hardly know this beauty by my side...

We are dancing, yet I am not wearing red. I am not wearing anything. Neither is my dance partner. And he does know me. We have known each other for years now. Yet this is the first time we have danced like this. He is one of my surrogate clients. We are not cheek to cheek but we are slow dancing, fingers intertwined, eyes smiling at one another. He is my partner for the afternoon.

When I arrived that day at his apartment, he was eager to tell me the surprise he had for me. He skipped saying hello and went right to his explanation.

"There are things I've never done. Because of my condition. Certain things that other people just do, and one of them is playing music for someone else. I've never played music for someone visiting me. I think people do that. They put on music they think the person would like." His words flowed quickly, not stopping between sentences, and then he paused suddenly, before continuing.

"I want to do that now."

"Of course. I would love to..." I began.

Before I could finish my sentence, he was showing me how he set up speakers to his laptop that is connected to his television. The speakers are sitting on a folding chair in the doorway of the bedroom, facing out towards the living room where we spend our time. We have to be careful walking to the bathroom through the bedroom as the wires from the speakers have created a trip hazard we must step over.

"I don't have those speakers other people have, that you don't need to plug in, so I had to do this. I have CDs but no CD player anymore. So I made a playlist on YouTube. I hope you like it."

My client was diagnosed many years ago with Asperger's syndrome, now referred to as a condition on the autism spectrum, although he doesn't use those terms. He says "my condition" and he doesn't want to dwell on it ever. But over the years he has shared how his condition prevented him from dating and having intimate relationships. With me he gets to practice. Someday he hopes to find a girlfriend. We recently started meeting at his apartment so he can experience what it could be like to bring a date or partner home.

The first time at his apartment he was eager to show me all of the options I had for something to drink in his fridge. After showing me, he told me to feel at home and I could have whatever I wanted. I thanked him for the options and for suggesting I make myself at home and help myself to a drink, but let him know that often hosts will offer to get the drink for their guests.

He understood right away. He started over and asked what I would like to drink and I said coconut water please. He asked if I wanted it in a mug or glass and I chose a glass, and he poured it for me and handed it to me. Everything we do together is an opportunity for him to learn social skills and to experience physical and emotional intimacy.

The music is new for us. When he started to play it, I suggested we dance. He suggested we do it without our clothes. I am the only woman he has ever been naked with and he likes to spend most of our two-hour session naked in order to make the most of the time we have. We enjoy talking, cuddling, eating (sometimes playfully off each other's bodies), we shower and wash each other and he brushes my hair afterwards. And once in a while we have sex.

But today we are dancing. The music on the playlist is from the 1980s, the music of both of our childhoods. The songs are as familiar to me as my own skin. I know all the words and I sing to him as he follows my rhythm and the movement of my body.

I've never seen you looking so gorgeous as you did tonight, I've never seen you shine so bright, you were amazing...

I move closer in and put my arms around his neck and rest my head on his shoulder. His hands are unsure where to go. I move them down to my waist. He is holding me close and I think of the prom he never attended, the dates he never went on, missed stolen kisses and groping on the corner or backseat of a car. For many of us who had that, it wasn't all perfect moments, far from it, but to never have had any of it seems cruel.

I can't give him back his teenage years, his twenties, thirties or forties. I can only be present with him now. Our naked bodies swaying happily to the sounds of our youth. I visualize pouring love into him, love he thought he would never have.

He still marvels that we are spending time together. "I can't believe I'm dancing with a beautiful naked lady," he says. At a certain point he had resigned himself to a sex life of pornography and secret crushes on female friends. He taught himself how to be a good friend. He had few friends as a child. As an adult he studied what it meant to be a friend and how to maintain connection. He works at it continually. He cares for his friends and he cares for me—although he will forget sometimes to ask how I'm doing or he might ask and then quickly start talking about himself before I finish my answer. We work on these skills. He also sees a therapist in between our sessions to help him process our work together. This is the surrogate partner therapy triadic model—working with a surrogate and a licensed therapist.

It was through a female friend that he found out about surrogate partner therapy. He asked if he could see her naked. "She said no," he told me, "but she didn't judge me. She stayed friends with me. She did some research and found out about surrogates."

He looks happy and remarks he is pleased he is doing well with the dancing, something he has very little experience with. I show him some disco moves and he spins me and brings me back in to face him. I once told him I felt safe with him and he said that was one of the nicest things anyone had ever said to him. At the time, I didn't realize the power of those words. He explained that as a child he sometimes did things that were upsetting to people and he felt people were afraid of him. Back then there was little understanding of autism and he was seen as a difficult child. In addition, his mother had mental health issues and she took out her frustration on him. He mostly doesn't talk about her, but when we first met, he told me how, at times, her stress would build up and she would go in a rage towards him.

"She would take me in a room and beat me with a stick. She would get physically tired and have to rest and catch her breath and then she would beat me again. She would say I was a terrible son. It was terrifying. She stopped when I was about ten because I was getting too big."

When he brought it up once in family therapy, she denied it and said he was a liar. He never talked about it again, until sharing with me and the therapist. He was sent to live in group homes for much of his childhood and teenage years. For a long time, he internalized his mother's words.

I've never seen so many people want to be there by your side,
And when you turned to me and smiled, it took my breath away...

We spend much of the session dancing with big smiles. We take snack breaks and talk about the music he chose. He shows me his CD collection. They are from whenever he has seen someone playing music out and about and he buys their CD to support them. They are all still wrapped in plastic as he doesn't have a CD player anymore. "I feel good about supporting the musicians," he says proudly. He very much wants to be a kind person and works at making decisions that show kindness.

We leave some time for our shower, which is one of our

favorite activities to share. In surrogate training, we practice having a silent sensual shower. In our sessions, he often talks a lot about his favorite things—science fiction movies and television shows. The shower quickly became a way to bring him to the moment and be present in his body, to feel sensation and to quiet his mind. In the shower, he stops talking. I shampoo his hair, taking time to slowly massage his scalp with my fingertips. His eyes close and he relaxes and sighs heavily as the hot water falls over him, washing the frothy shampoo down his body. Then he does my hair and we soap up each other's bodies, taking extra care to caress genitals, keeping it sexy, and finish with some oil. We are happy, relaxed, slippery and clean and I lean into him, sometimes standing in front of him, both of us facing forward and he wraps his arms around me and caresses my breasts while I wiggle my butt playfully against his genitals.

And I have never had such a feeling, Such a feeling of complete and utter love, as I do tonight...

When we first met, he brought a measuring tape and ruler with him. He wanted to know the length of my perineum and the size of my clitoris. I told him we would not be undressing at our first session, likely not for several sessions. He explained to me he was fascinated by the vulva.

"It is like a foreign planet to me. Someplace I have never been, never thought I would get to visit, but I have studied extensively."

Far more than being sexual with me, he wanted to examine me, to understand the secret world he had been missing. When he finally did see my vulva, he asked, "Have I really left the earth's atmosphere and seen a vulva?" as he struggled with deciding if it counted, since his first glimpse of it wasn't close up. He decided it counted and he made a note of the date. He eventually got a close-up look but by then we had moved through many exercises of getting to know each other's bodies and he was less interested in the exact length of the various parts, although still fascinated by them.

He admitted that perhaps he was still in the playing doctor phase of his sexual development since he never had that as a child. "This is all new to me," he would say. "I feel like a child." I told him at one point that when I was with him, I experienced him as a man, not a boy. He said that was the second nicest thing someone had said to him in a long time.

I have had many clients who have had a lack of healthy mothering and I can sense how they crave a nurturing mother figure. Sometimes just holding them and caressing their face feels like desperately needed medicine. I acknowledge this desire while remembering that they are here to learn to be adult lovers, to be a partner to someone. In many healthy adult intimate relationships, there is some degree of that craving for pure nurturance. Sometimes we all just want to be held by "mommy" or "daddy." We also want a partner who can show up as an adult. I keep the focus on how this person can learn to be a good lover and a good partner to someone.

In surrogate partner therapy, we create a relationship. It is real. There can be real feelings. The feelings of tenderness I have for this client are real. But the relationship is not limitless. It has boundaries. The goal of the work is for the client to graduate and go out and find the love and intimacy they are seeking, with someone who is fully available for that. If a client expresses feelings of love for me, I invoke Maude in the film *Harold and Maude*. That's wonderful, go and love some more.

We talk about what he is looking for in a girlfriend. "I don't want someone with my condition. Just because two people are autistic doesn't mean they have things in common. I want someone to accept me as I am," he says emphatically.

At our next session with music, he is excited to offer me "wine" in a wine glass. It is really juice, but he wants to practice serving someone wine. We clink our glasses and toast to a beautiful date. Soon our glasses are empty and we are getting undressed, ready for our next dance.

I never will forget the way you look tonight...

The lady in red, the lady in red,

The lady in red, my lady in red...

CHAPTER 19
HOLDING HANDS

Maya

Ruth was a lesbian who had only recently come out to herself at the age of 62. She had never had any wanted sexual touch in her life and had never been sexual with a woman. She was my first surrogate partner client. We were early on in our process, just getting to know each other.

At the beginning of surrogate partner therapy, we often start with a hand caress and face caress, using the method of sensate focus, but for Ruth, even this was a challenge. It was her idea to use a scarf in between our hands for her to feel safe enough to touch.

"I see you brought your scarf," I smile at Ruth. We are seated close together on the couch in my office, our legs almost touching.

"I thought we could use it for touching hands," she replies, her eyes looking away for a moment.

"Yes, let's give it a try," I reassure her. "Are you comfortable with me sitting here? This close?"

"Yes, I think so," she pauses. "Yes, I am," she states more confidently, but still looks nervous. I can hear her breathing quicken.

"Okay. Should we take some deep breaths before we start?"

Ruth nods her head.

We close our eyes and start to breathe deeply. I open one eye and sneak a glance at Ruth to see if she is okay.

I speak softly. "Keep breathing, feel your body relax, feel your weight sink into the couch, let everything go…"

I open my eyes after a few more breaths and see that Ruth looks more at ease.

"Okay, let's open our eyes."

I smile at her and she is smiling back. "Are we ready?" I ask.

"Yes, I am ready," she replies with a giggle. I giggle a little too.

I take the scarf and place it over Ruth's hand which is resting on her own thigh. Very slowly and gently I place my hand over the scarf, gazing down at our hands. I lift my eyes to Ruth's face. She does not look relaxed anymore.

"Is it okay?" I ask.

"Yes," she says, and her eyes start to well up.

We sit in silence for a few moments. Her body starts to relax again.

"What if we try with my hand on top?" Ruth suggests.

"Sure, let's try."

We rearrange so my hand is resting on my own leg, the scarf on top and then Ruth's hand over the scarf.

"I don't know. This is scarier," she says.

"Why scarier?"

"What if I hurt you?" she asks.

"I trust you." I look directly into her eyes. "I feel safe with you."

Ruth's eyes well up again.

"I just realized that in my family, hands were for hurting," she says.

My face softens as I nod my head slowly. Ruth removes her hand and turns away. Then looks back at me.

"It sounds as if you are carrying that pain and fear with you still," I say.

She nods and looks at her hands.

"I know I am safe with you. I am not worried about you hurting me. Do you feel safe with me?" I ask.

She looks at me and nods her head.

"I do. I feel safe here," she says.

"We will go slowly. There is no rush. You get to decide the pace."

Ruth swallows nervously. "Let's try again," she suggests. I nod my head.

"What if we do palms facing each other?" I ask.

"Okay, let's try," she says.

"Do you want to be top or bottom?" I raise my eyebrow and grin at the sexual reference.

"I don't know if I'm a top or a bottom," Ruth giggles.

"We shall see...all in good time..." I smile at her.

Ruth takes a deep breath and sighs it out.

"I'll be bottom," she suggests.

Ruth puts her hand on her own lap face up and using her other hand places the scarf on top. I place my hand slowly and gently on top of the scarf.

We both look down at our hands.

Ruth's breath quickens. She starts to move her hand a little, gradually opening her fingers. I respond by following Ruth's lead.

I am moving my hand along with hers.

Ruth starts to curl her fingers around the scarf, around my hand.

Her breathing gets louder and deeper. I smile and start to curl my fingers as well.

"We are holding hands," I say.

"We are holding hands. I am holding hands. I am..."

Ruth's eyes well up as her words trail off. I smile at Ruth, hoping she can feel all of the love and compassion I am pouring into her.

"Are you okay? Is it okay?" I ask.

Ruth's facial expression becomes serious.

"She bent my fingers back. She hurt me."

"Who did?" I ask quietly, feeling the heaviness of what she is sharing.

"My mother. I had to go to the hospital. No one talked about it."

Our eyes meet.

"I'm so sorry you went through that. I can't imagine."

"Why would she do that to a child? Her child?" She knows she is asking a question without an answer.

"You didn't deserve that. No one does," I say, hoping my eyes are conveying the depth of compassion I feel for her.

"I know. I know that now," Ruth says.

Suddenly she looks determined.

"You are brave," I say.

"I don't know if I'm brave, but I'm tired of being alone. No more scarf," Ruth says emphatically.

She grabs the scarf and tosses it away. She takes my hand in her own.

"Now we are holding hands," she says. "I want this."

I smile big at her. "Wow, we are really holding hands. I do think you're brave. This isn't easy."

"You're right. It's not easy. Thank you. Thank you for being here when I needed you. I don't know how else I would have... I mean how can you have a relationship with someone if you can't even hold hands?"

I nod my head.

"And sex, I can't even imagine..."

Ruth takes a deep breath and smiles. I smile back at her.

"Well, that's why you're here. So you don't have to just imagine. It can be a reality. One step at a time. No rush. A slow journey."

"I'm ready. I want a relationship. I want sex! I can say that now."

Ruth looks energized. I hold her gaze.

"Thank you for trusting me. We will get there," I say, hoping to instill confidence.

Ruth nods her head.

"What now?" she asks, looking down at our hands.

"We could explore each other's hands. Using sensate focus. Touch for your own pleasure. Touch my hand in a way that feels good to you."

Ruth begins to run her hand over my hand, moving slowly, exploring the spaces between my fingers, her palm.

"Your hand is soft," she smiles at me.

"Thank you. Yours too. May I explore?"

Ruth hesitates for a moment. "Yes, you may," she gives permission.

I close my eyes and begin to explore Ruth's hand with my own. Using the back of my hand, I move it slowly inside her palm. I then move my fingers in between her fingers. Ruth closes her eyes and lets out a sigh. Her body is relaxing. She is enjoying the touch.

"This is good. I like this," she says, a little surprised at herself.

"I do too," I say, and I mean it.

"From here, we will move on to other body parts," I say and then pause. I realize we have just hit a milestone and I shouldn't move too quickly.

"When you're ready for that," I clarify.

"What body part is next?" she asks.

"Actually face," I say, "a face caress."

Ruth's expression tells me she wants to know more.

I lift my free hand up to my cheek and fold my fingers in and gently stroke. My head tilts slightly in the direction of my hand as I slowly caress myself. For a moment my eyes close. Then I open them slowly and look at Ruth. My hand moves down from my cheek and lands below my collarbone. I take a deep breath and lightly pat my skin and then begin to twirl my hair in my hand as I grin at Ruth.

"Are you flirting with me?" Ruth asks, expectantly.

"I think I might be..."

Ruth looks happy.

"This is fun."

"I hope so. It should be fun."

"But I'm still so scared of having sex with a woman."

"Trust the process. By the time we get there, you will be ready. Because if you're not ready, we won't go there. I will show you the path, but you set the pace."

"Okay. Part of me is ready, sooo ready. I want touch. I want love."

"It's what we all need—love and affection."

"May I touch your face?" Ruth asks.

"You may." I sit up straight and offer my face to her, eyes closed. Ruth lifts her hand to my cheek and begins to caress it. I open my eyes.

We are looking at each other with love, with longing, with sweetness. For a moment, nothing else exists. The couch, the lamp, my office walls all disappear. We are only aware of each other's energy. Ruth feels it.

"It's just two people. Two people together. I mean, how can it be so...? How can it feel so...?" Ruth's voice trails off.

"So simple. But so powerful."

"You know at first I thought this was just going to be about sex."

I grin at her.

"Sex is never just about sex. It's so much more. Just wait. You're gonna love the more."

Ruth grins back at me.

"I already do," she says.

CONTRIBUTORS

Eva Alio helped clients who were ready to restore their ability to authentically and intimately connect. She did this with gentle trauma integration guidance, deep caring, relaxation, mindfulness and pleasure practices. For these sessions she combined knowledge from professional trainings and personal life experience to meet clients where they were at. At the time of publication, Eva Alio is engaged in spiritual pursuits and not accepting clients. To see where she is today, try www.EvaAlio.com.

A.M. Ament is a clinician with roots in street culture and sex work in many US cities since the mid-90s. They are an award-winning theorist, former music journalist, paramedic, poet and all over attention deficit hyperactivity disorder (ADHD) superstar, seeking to stop harm in institutional settings. They founded their practice, Stardust Therapy, in Seattle in 2019, using the social model to work with marginalized people in marginalized communities. Their special interests include shoegaze music, disability justice, bodily autonomy and biopsychology. They identify as an intersex, hard femme, disabled weirdo with a high capacity for love in a cruel and unjust world.

Fariba Arabghani is a Black, Indigenous Person of Color (BI-POC), queer, neurodivergent, kinky and polyamorous marketing professional turned board-certified sexologist, AASECT CSE, and educator. She is a graduate of the Kinsey Institute's Human Sexuality Intensive Program, is certified by Johns Hopkins University in psychological first aid, and is currently pursuing American Association of Sexuality Educators, Counselors and Therapists (AASECT) Sexuality Educator Certification. Her work focuses on the intersectionality of marginalized identities, alternative sexuality and social justice. Informed by her personal and professional experiences, she provides cultural competency consulting to clinical, academic and research settings, and facilitates workshops on sexuality justice and inclusion. Her expertise has been featured in several publications, including *Cosmopolitan*, *Glamour*, *Kinkly* and *Men's Health*, and in LiveJasmin's "Life in Red" docuseries.

JoJo Bear is a native-born New Yorker, a half Puerto Rican and Sicilian, poly, queer bear. He is a somatic sex and intimacy guide, sacred intimate and coach in the San Francisco Bay Area—mentor to sex workers, intimacy coaches and fellow facilitators. JoJo is part of the faculty of the Body Electric School and teaches for the School of Consent. His passion is to help gay, bisexual, transgender and queer men get out of their heads and into their bodies. He lives with his husband Ken and two dogs, Rocket and Whiskey.

e.b. cotenord is a Chicago-based professional dream girl, a sex worker, writer and the host of The eXXXistential Podcast. Her creative endeavors serve as explorations into her experiences navigating society as a current sex worker and recovering addict. e.b. is a single mother raising two teenagers as well as three mischievous rabbits. She seeks to help humanize marginalized communities by writing about her life as an adult entertainer and suburban mom in recovery. She can be found on X @ebcotenord.

Victoria Angel Heart, M.Ed, CMT-P, is a passionate pleasure permissionary, dedicated to empowering folx to embrace intimacy within themselves, their relationships and with all of life. She's the founder of Tap into Freedom & Psychedelic EFT. Alongside her work as a plant medicine and embodied intimacy guide, she weaves her original "hypnotic hymns" and empowerment anthems as a permissionary of song and full embodied expression of feeling. Victoria organizes engaging music and intimacy events regularly throughout the Bay Area. She believes in the power of the transformative healing that occurs when we connect with ourselves and embody intimacy, together.

Sadie Hudson is a full-service sex worker based in Vancouver, British Columbia, Canada. Prior to sex work, Sadie held a variety of jobs, ranging from research to human services to construction, and in her early thirties, completed a BA (Honors) at a Canadian university. She feels that sex work is a calling and that her resonance with the work is innate to her sexuality itself. She established sovereignsexworkers.com, a blog about the business and craft of sex work, designed for the career enrichment of sex workers. When she is not writing or seeing clients, she is studying astrology, doing pilates or yoga, or appreciating the beauty of our natural environment.

Daddy Lance is a sacred intimate, surrogate partner and massage therapist based out of St Pete, Florida. He began his journey into the erotic healing arts in 2008 after leaving his retail management job to find deeper purpose in life. He regards his work as deeply spiritual and believes that vulnerability is the key to living the most wholehearted life possible. Though he mostly works with cisgender men, he has worked with transmen as well and cis and transwomen and is passionate about working with people with disabilities.

Tracy Lee is a sexual visionary guide. She began this work after friends kept turning to her for relationship and intimacy advice. She has an intense curiosity for learning and exploration; her deep presence, coupled with childlike playfulness, helps clients feel safe and at ease. She has training in mindfulness, Reiki healing, pelvic massage, tantra and somatic therapy. In sessions, she addresses what you think and how that affects what you feel. This combination helps clients to feel free and accept themselves without societal guilt or shame, and to enjoy pleasure longer, with more sensation and intensity. Her website is www.sessionswithtracy.com.

Maya is a certified surrogate partner who was trained by the International Professional Surrogates Association (IPSA) in 2016. She feels it is a privilege to join clients on their journey of sexual awakening and healing through surrogate partner therapy.

Mehdi has worked for over 25 years as a psychotherapist and has specialized in trauma and sexuality. He has graduate degrees in counseling psychology and art therapy, and training in sandplay therapy, sexological bodywork and somatic sex education. He lives on Vancouver Island on the west coast of Canada. Mehdi's approach, Perfect Touch, is based on connecting people with their authentic self and pleasure, and helping them find creative solutions towards consensual and pleasurable relationships with self and others. His clientele include adults with histories of trauma and couples with sex and relationship challenges. He can be found at https://thetouchingcure.com.

Don Shewey is a writer, therapist and pleasure activist in New York City. As a journalist and critic, he has published three books about theater and hundreds of articles for the *New York Times*, *Esquire*, *Rolling Stone* and other publications. He has chronicled his psycho-sexual-spiritual adventures in *The Paradox of Porn: Notes on Gay Male Sexual Culture* and in essays for numerous anthologies, including *The Politics of Manhood* and *The Queerest Art: Essays on Lesbian and Gay Theater*. His most recent book is *Daddy Lover God: A Sacred Intimate Journey*. An archive of his writing is available online at www.donshewey.com.

Natasha Strange is a professional dominant, dungeon owner, BDSM educator, published author, an aspiring cult leader and a wicked minx, with nearly 30 years' experience in the world of kink and BDSM. As an educator, she excels at creating approachable spaces to explore scary, intimidating things through the use of puns and laughter. Her book, *Kink for the Curious*, is a whimsical activity book with puzzles and color pages, as well as solid information about kink and BDSM. As a dominant, she feeds on nervous energy and enjoys escaping with her playthings into their darkest fantasies.

Court Vox is a certified sex and intimacy coach surrogate partner intern and sacred intimate based in Los Angeles, California. He is a member of the World Association of Sex Coaches, and founder of The Body Vox. He is a guide for a vast spectrum of individuals and those in relationship/s seeking more in their erotic and intimate lives. When it comes to human connection and sexuality, some are beginning their journey while others have been pursuing erotic education and experiences for years. Court works gently with first-timers, as well as offering uncommon experiences to some of the world's most well-known sex educators and change-makers across multiple fields and disciplines. Court has become known for offering private, highly customized, exclusive experiences and he travels extensively hosting and teaching workshops for all bodies, genders and orientations. Court is also part of an elite team of sex educators that created the celebrated program for women, Back to the Body, which runs retreats all across the globe.

Wendy is a sexuality educator, who worked as an escort while she was in graduate school. Her experience opened her eyes to the complexity of reasons why men may seek out sex work, and increased her compassion for men in general, something she did not expect.

BD White is an educator, activist and mother, loving and living in the beautiful North Bay area in California. She is currently pursuing an advanced degree in the field of psychology. Her disciplines include transpersonal/depth psychology and social psychology, with a research focus on masculinity and its interactions with many aspects of the human experience, from relationships to social justice and policy.

Emme Witt-Eden is a Los Angeles-based writer with bylines in *Vice*, *Business Insider*, *The Daily Dot*, *Yahoo Life*, *Cosmo*, *Giddy* and *MetroUK*. A former professional dominatrix turned kink consultant, her insights have been featured in publications such as *Women's Health*, *The Daily Beast*, *Mashable*, *MEL Magazine*, *Dame* and *Kinkly*, helping to demystify once-taboo sexual practices. More information: www.emmewitt.com.

EDITOR

Remi Newman is a sexuality educator and writer, living in Northern California. She has a master's degree in sexuality education from New York University and over 20 years' experience working as a sexuality educator and counselor. She is the proud mama of a teenage son, several naughty kitties and the occasional crayfish. You can find her writing at Blog. Kinkly.com.

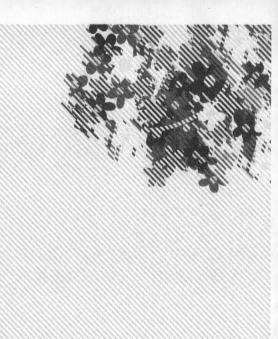

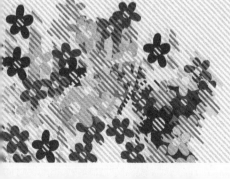